Parotidectomy

General Editor, Wolfe Surgical Atlases:
William F. Walker, DSc, ChM, FRCS (Edin. and England), FRS (Edin.).

Single Surgical Procedures 1

A Colour Atlas of

Parotidectomy

Michael Hobsley
TD, PH.D, M.CHIR, FRCS
Professor of Surgery
Department of Surgical Studies
Middlesex Hospital
London W1

Wolfe Medical Publications Ltd

Copyright © Michael Hobsley, 1983
Published by Wolfe Medical Publications Ltd, 1983
Printed by Royal Smeets Offset b.v.,
Weert, Netherlands
ISBN 0 7234 1006 2

This book is one of the titles in the series of
Wolfe Single Surgical Procedures, a series which
will eventually cover some 200 titles.
   If you wish to be kept informed of new
additions to the series and receive details of our
other titles, please write to
Wolfe Medical Publications Ltd, Wolfe House,
3 Conway Street, London W1P 6HE.

A few of the other titles in preparation in the
Single Surgical Procedures series

Inguinal Hernias & Hydroceles in Infants & Children
Traditional Meniscectomy
Surgery for Pancreatic & Associated Carcinomata
Subtotal Thyroidectomy
Boari Bladder-Flap Procedure
Treatment of Carpal Tunnel Syndrome
Surgery for Varicose Veins
Anterior Resection of Rectum
Resection of Aortic Aneurysm
Modified Radical Mastectomy
Total Gastrectomy
Ileo-Rectal Anastomosis
Pre-Prosthetic Oral Surgery
Surgery for Undescended Testes
Techniques of Nerve Grafting and Repair
Surgery for Dupuytren's Contracture
Arthrodesis of the Ankle
Surgery for Congenital Dislocation of the Hip
Common Operations of the Foot
Femoral and Tibial Osteotomy
Maxillo-Facial Traumatology
Surgery for Chondromalacia Patellae
Stabilisation for Extensive Spinal Injury
Laminectomy
Gall Bladder Cholecystectomy
Repair of Prolapsed Rectum
Proctocolectomy
Resection of Oesophagus
Splenectomy
Thyroid Lobectomy

Contents

Dedication

The modern operation of parotidectomy with conservation of the facial nerve has gradually evolved since about 1940 as a result of the work of Janes in Canada and Hamilton Bailey in the UK. Later important contributions were made by Redon in France, and particularly by a great surgeon and gentleman who taught the author almost all he knows about parotidectomy, and a good deal of what he has learned about everything else.

This book is dedicated in all humility to the memory of that man, David Patey.

Michael Hobsley

Acknowledgements

This book could not have been prepared without the enthusiasm and skill of Mr R.R. Phillips, FIIP, FRPS, Head of the Department of Medical Photography, The Middlesex Hospital, who was responsible for the photographs.

I am also grateful to Mrs Judith Sinclair and Miss Susannah Wright for typing the manuscript.

Introduction

The surgical removal of the parotid salivary gland is complicated by the presence within the gland of the trunk and branches of the facial (7th cranial) nerve. Destruction of this nerve produces a paralysis of the ipsilateral half of the face with a consequent inability to corrugate the forehead, raise the eyebrow, close the eye, blow or whistle, or pull the corner of the mouth laterally. The lack of blinking of the eye results in profuse weeping of the eye and a tendency to conjunctivitis, while the paralysis of the buccinator muscle in the cheek results in food collecting in the cheek during chewing. The attempt to smile pulls the mouth over to the unaffected side. The only indication for subjecting a patient to this mutilation is that neoplastic disease cannot otherwise be adequately treated.

Parotidectomy can be classified in a number of different ways.

With reference to the facial nerve, parotidectomy may be either *radical* – in which case the nerve is sacrificed; *conservative* – in which case all main branches of the facial nerve are preserved; or *semi-conservative* – in which case one or more, but not all, of the main branches are sacrificed. Fine nervous twigs which are present in addition to the main branches, or connect across from one main branch to another, can be divided without altering the designation of an operation as conservative because there seems to be no risk of permanent facial paralysis in those circumstances. There are six main branches: the *temporal branch* to the forehead, the *zygomatic branch* to the orbit, and usually the upper *buccal branch* to the upper half of the cheek and nose arise from the main upper division of the nerve, while from the main lower subdivision of the nerve arise the *platysmal branch* to the neck, the *mandibular branch* to the angle of the mouth, and (usually) the *lower buccal branch* to the lower half of the cheek and nose and the upper lip. The arrangement of the buccal branches in particular is very variable; sometimes both arise from the upper division, sometimes both from the lower division, and sometimes there may be one or more extra buccal branches. As long as two buccal branches are preserved, one running towards the upper half of the cheek and one running towards the lip, the operation can be classed as a conservative parotidectomy.

Parotidectomy can also be classed according to the extent of tissue removed, as *superficial, total, deep*, or as part of a more extensive resection. If in dissecting forwards the branches of the facial nerve as much of the parotid tissue superficial to the nerve is removed as possible, the operation is a *conservative superficial parotidectomy*. If after the nerves have been dissected forwards and the superficial parotid removed, the nerves are then elevated from their bed and the remainder of the parotid salivary gland deep to the nerves removed from under them (but preserving the continuity of the nerves), the operation is a *total conservative parotidectomy*. Occasionally it may be possible, having reflected the superficial parotid forwards, to remove the deep part of the parotid without actually removing the superficial part: such an operation would be a *deep conservative parotidectomy* but it is not recommended because of the risk of fistula formation.

Total radical parotidectomy may also be a part of a far more major resection for cancer, perhaps with block dissection of the cervical lymph nodes, resection of the posterior third of the hemimandible, resection of the zygoma and of the external auditory meatus. Such operations bear little relation to the painstaking conservative operation with dissection and preservation of the facial nerve.

Before embarking on parotidectomy for a lump, the surgeon should always warn the patient that it might be necessary to sacrifice the facial nerve, or one or more of its branches, if a satisfactory clearance is to be achieved.

Permission to sacrifice the facial nerve must always be obtained (see page 91).

Indications for parotidectomy

The most common indication for parotidectomy is a lump in the parotid region which is well demarcated, slowly growing, and has produced no evidence of interference with the facial nerve. Eighty per cent of such lesions turn out to be a neoplasm of parotid tissue, and 75 per cent of those turn out to be a pleomorphic salivary adenoma. This tumour, in common with other salivary adenomas (monomorphic adenomas), is benign in the sense that metastases are almost unrecorded, but shows a remarkable ability to produce local recurrence if cells from the tumour are shed and become implanted in the wound. Thus, not one but two major considerations dominate the operation for a lump in the parotid region: not only must the nerve be preserved (unless the lump is actually growing into the nerve), but also a margin of normal tissue must be maintained around the lump at all stages of the dissection.

The only other indication which is at all common is longstanding inflammation, usually caused by calculous disease but occasionally by other causes of unknown aetiology such as Sjögren's syndrome. In such patients the dissection of the branches of the facial nerve may be more difficult because of inflammatory adhesions to surrounding tissue, but the important problem of keeping away from a lump and yet preserving the branches of the facial nerve do not arise. The illustrations of parotidectomy in this book are therefore derived from operations for a lump in the parotid region. No one operation can illustrate all the points that require comment and so three operations will be shown.

Parotidectomy as part of a more extensive procedure has already been mentioned.

Total conservative parotidectomy

Fifteen per cent of parotid tumours lie deep to the facial nerve, but in most such patients physical examination cannot reveal whether the lump is superficial or deep to the nerve. It follows that the surgeon must be prepared to perform a total conservative parotidectomy if he embarks upon an operation for a lump in the parotid region. No matter how superficial and mobile the lump appears to be, it might still be deep to the facial nerve.

Very occasionally, it may be possible to diagnose that the lump is in the deep portion of the gland by the fact that it bulges into the lateral wall of the pharynx in the region of the tonsillar fossa.

1 and 2 Lump in front and below attachment of pinna. A 35-year-old man complained of a lump just in front and below the lower anterior attachment of the pinna to the face. These lateral and anterior views show that the lump was by no means prominent in this region, and several observers decided it was a lymph node of no important significance.

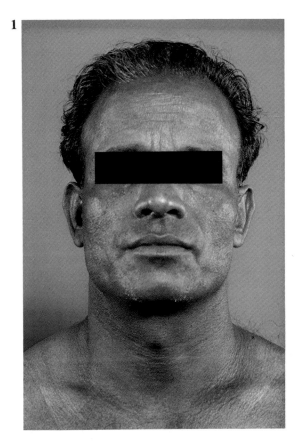
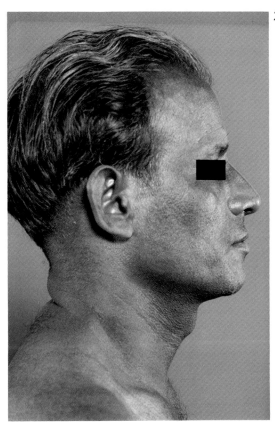

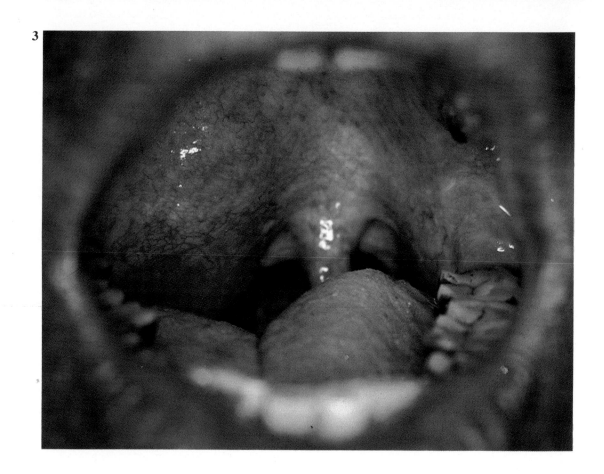

3 Parotid gland tumour. However, on looking inside the mouth, the reddened wall of the right side of the pharynx can be seen clearly bulging towards the midline, because of the presence of the tumour in the deep part of the parotid gland.

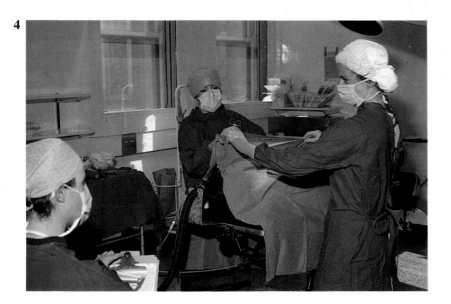

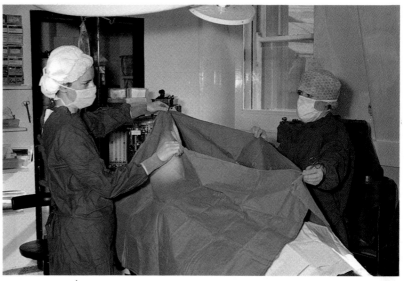

4 Skin preparation and towelling. The patient has been anaesthetised (induction with intravenous sodium thiopentone, intubation with a nasal endotracheal tube, nitrous oxide, oxygen and halothane). Further details of preliminary stages will be found in **5** to **8**. Skin preparation has been performed and towelling-up is now in process. A white paper drape has been laid across the chest and abdomen, reaching from the suprasternal notch above, to the pelvis below. Two assistants hold the sterile side towels which have been fastened together at each end with a towel clip. Each assistant holds a towel clip in her left hand and the middle of the edge of the towel nearest to her with her right hand. Placing the side towels first protects the sterile gowns of the assistants from contamination by non-sterile surfaces of the operating table or the patient.

5 Another view of towelling-up. Another angle of the towelling-up process shown in **4**. Note the position of the anaesthetist and his apparatus in a prolongation from the head-end of the operating table. Some anaesthetists prefer to have their apparatus near the foot of the table, but I find towelling-up easier with the anaesthetist in the position shown. This still leaves room for a first assistant to sit on the side of the lesion between the operator and the anaesthetist and for a second assistant to stand opposite the surgeon.

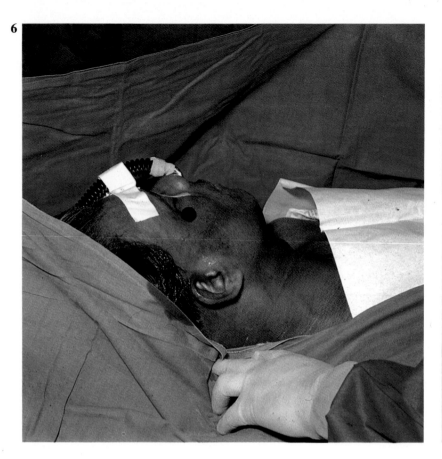

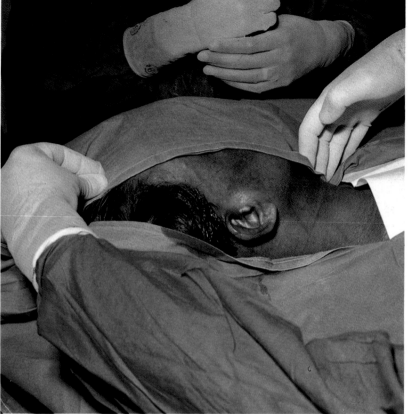

6 Correct placing of right towel. The towel on the patient's right being placed in its correct position, well posterior to the ear. Hair has been shaved so that there is a hairless area around the pinna and well posteriorly down the right side of the neck. The white paper drape is seen at its upper end in this figure, and more details of the nasal endotracheal tube and its support. Note that any taping applied by the anaesthetist must stop short of the operative area. The anaesthetist has protected the eyes against injury from antiseptic lotions used in cleaning the skin by filling them with a lubricant paste and taping the right eye shut.

7 Correct placing of left towel. The left side towel is now being placed accurately in the position desired. The face is exposed as far forwards as the cheek at the anterior border of the masseter muscle. Some surgeons advocate leaving a corner of the eye exposed so that it can by its twitching give warning that the facial nerve is being stimulated by the dissection. However, there is no difficulty in seeing twitching of the facial muscles by their effect on the close-fitting overlying towels; leaving the eye exposed incurs an unnecessary risk of damage from blood or other liquids during the operation.

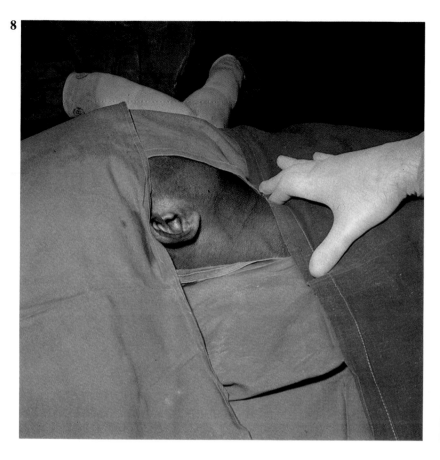

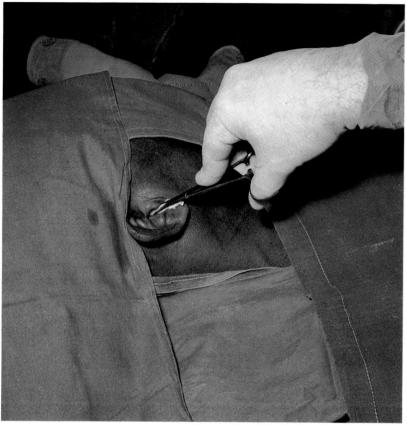

8 Placement of upper towel and long sheet. A small upper towel and a long sheet coming up towards the lower margin of the wound have now been placed. The area of skin exposed extends from the zygoma above to the clavicle below.

9 Protection of eardrum. The external ear has to be left exposed because the incision and dissection proceed very close to its margins. To avoid blood or other liquid collecting in the external auditory meatus, with the possibility of an induced inflammatory reponse, a twist of cottonwool is inserted in the meatus with a pair of artery forceps that are then discarded as contaminated.

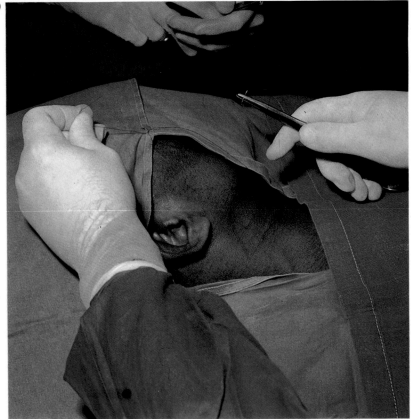

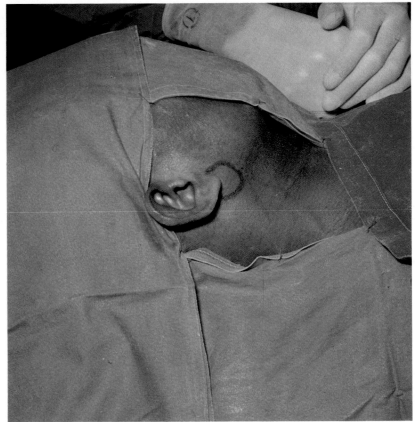

10 Sewing of towels. The towels are sewn accurately in position, the curved needle taking a bite through the patient's skin as well as through each towel. Stitching with 2–0 silk does not seem to produce keloid scarring, whereas towel clips can produce this complication. Adhesive strips for fixing the towel accurately in position would probably be a satisfactory alternative but the author finds stitching particularly convenient.

11 Use of blue dye as marker. As already mentioned, the lump in this patient was not obvious to ordinary inspection. To enable the reader to understand more clearly the relationship of the incision and the dissection to the palpable borders of the lump, a blue dye has been used to mark out those borders. Note in particular that in this view the lump seems to be fairly close to the lower anterior corner of the attachment of the pinna to the face. Note the obvious border of the lower edge of the mandible in this illustration. It lies at about the lower border of the lump. This may make it easier to appreciate the position of the first part of the incision shown in **12**.

12 Standard incision of parotidectomy. This is an S-shaped cervico-mastoid-facial incision, but the author finds it's best to make this incision in three separate portions starting from below and moving upwards. Thus when the cervical incision has been made all bleeding can be stopped before going on to the mastoid incision and so on. This prevents the surgeon's view of the lower part of the wound being obliterated by blood draining downwards from the upper parts of the wound.

The cervical part of the incision has been made in this illustration. It lies in the upper skin crease of the neck, which is at a much lower level than the mandible. **11** shows how the lower border of the mandible lay near the lower border of the lump; **12** demonstrates how the incision lies about three-fingers' breadth below the lower border of the lump. The posterior end of the incision is at a point vertically below where the pinna at its anteroinferior margin meets the face, while anteriorly the incision is carried forward to just in front of the external jugular vein. The incision has been deepened through skin and platysma and the first landmark identified – the great auricular nerve. At least 7 cm of this nerve is dissected as shown. If possible its upward course should be dissected until it starts to separate into branches, but that was not possible in this patient, because the dissection would have led one too close to the region of the lump itself.

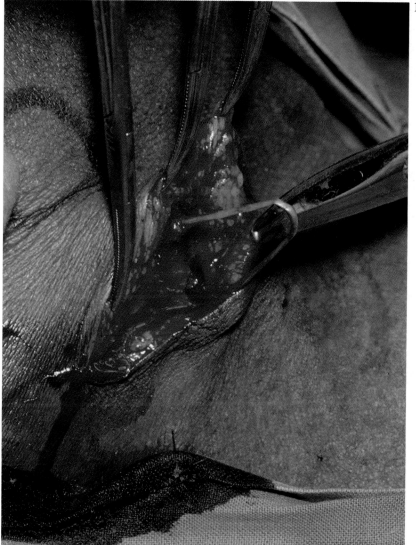

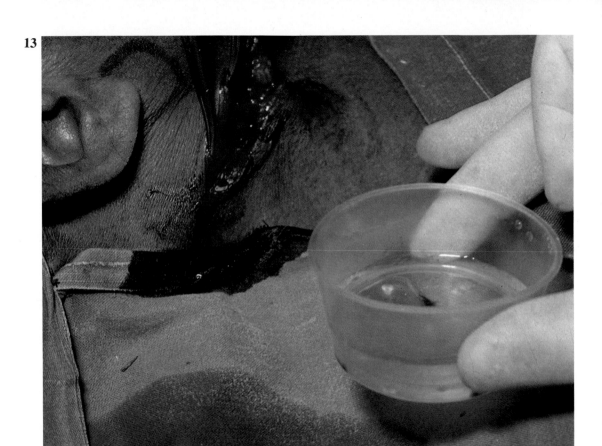

13 **Branches of auricular nerve.** The great auricular nerve is often in two branches, a smaller anterior and a larger posterior. It is occasionally feasible to attempt to preserve the smaller anterior branch, but the larger posterior (the only branch identified in this patient) cannot be preserved if an adequate removal of parotid tissue is to be performed. Therefore the author makes a virtue of necessity and excises a long segment of dissected nerve to keep in a bowl of isotonic saline until the end of the operation. Should it have been necessary to cut out a segment of facial nerve, whether branch or trunk, the segment of great auricular nerve can be used to bridge the defect as a so-called cable graft.

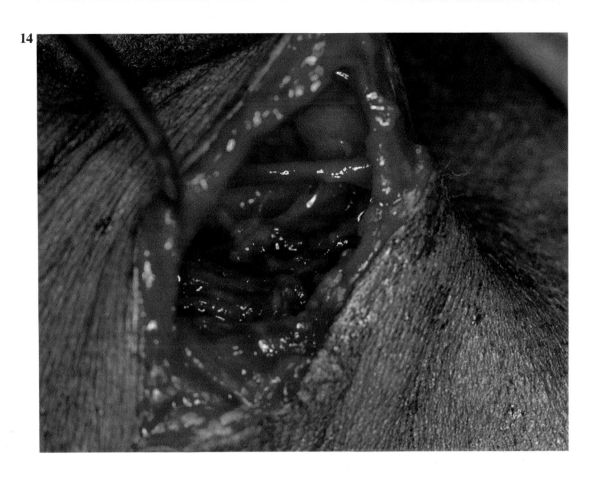

14 Exposure of sternomastoid muscle. Artery forceps on the subcutaneous tissue of the upper flap hold it upwards (see also **12**) and the dissection of the lower flap (i.e. keeping well away from the lump) is now deepened to expose the second landmark, the anterior border of the sternomastoid muscle. This can be seen as dark brown tissue running horizontally across this view. Lying above it is the exposed external jugular vein: it is not usually necessary to dissect this vein free at this early stage of the operation, but in this particular patient the vein lay very close to the anterior border of the sternomastoid and so it was dissected free to prevent accidental damage to it. This vein will be tied at a later stage of the operation but the author prefers not to tie it now if possible, in case the destruction of its drainage increases venous bleeding from the operative field during the dissection.

Deep to the anterior border of the sternomastoid, the posterior belly of the digastric and the stylohyoid are sometimes in their turn demonstrated at this stage of the dissection, but it was not found convenient to do so in the present case.

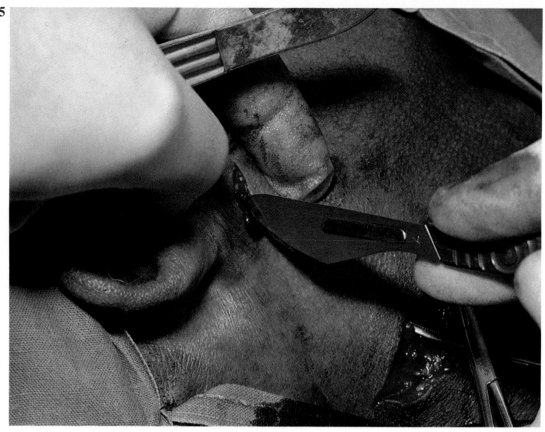

15   Cervico-mastoid-facial incision. The mastoid part of the cervico-mastoid-facial incision is next made. It runs from the anteroinferior point of attachment of the pinna to the face in the posterior and inferior direction to meet the posterior end of the cervical incision. It is absolutely imperative that the knife should not cut into the lump. Note how the surgeon's left index finger is pushing the lump forwards to bring it away from the knife blade. If a lump were even more inferior and posterior, it would be necessary to take the incision even further backwards so as to avoid cutting straight down on to the lump. It would be a tragedy if the depth of cut were misjudged and the knife cut into the tumour at this early stage of the operation.

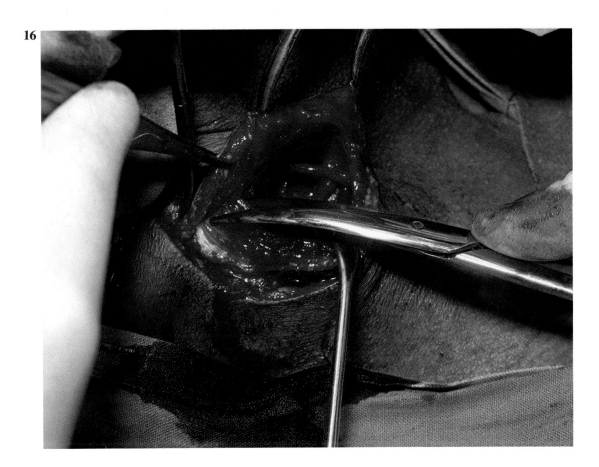

16 The anterior border of the sternomastoid is now followed upwards to its origin at the mastoid process. During this procedure the anterior flap of skin becomes to some extent elevated, but exercise great care to ensure that the parotid lump is pushed forward, should it be close to the anterior border of the sternomastoid. If necessary, and rather than possibly cutting into the lump, a few fibres of sternomastoid are left on the side of the lump (see **17**).

17 Exposure of digastric and stylohyoid muscles. Either earlier (see **14**) or now, the dissection in front of the sternomastoid muscle is deepened to expose the posterior belly of the digastric muscle and the stylohyoid muscle. To locate these muscles, it is essential to concentrate attention as posteriorly as possible, near the origin of the sternomastoid muscle from the mastoid process. In this illustration, the curved artery forceps is pointing at the posterior belly of the digastric running away from the surgeon towards the midline of the neck. The further the patient's head is turned to the side opposite the tumour, the more difficult it is to find this muscle because it is being stretched away from the surgeon. The head should therefore only be turned sufficiently to the opposite side to make access to the superficial part of the neck reasonably easy (see later, **61**).

The stylohyoid muscle is deep to the posterior belly of the digastric but has not yet been identified in this illustration. Note that the anterior skin flap, being held upwards with the dissecting forceps, contains a few muscle fibres of the sternomastoid which have been left in place to protect the lump.

17

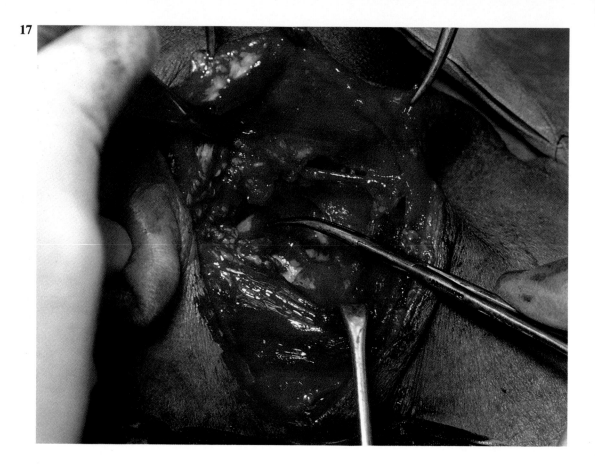

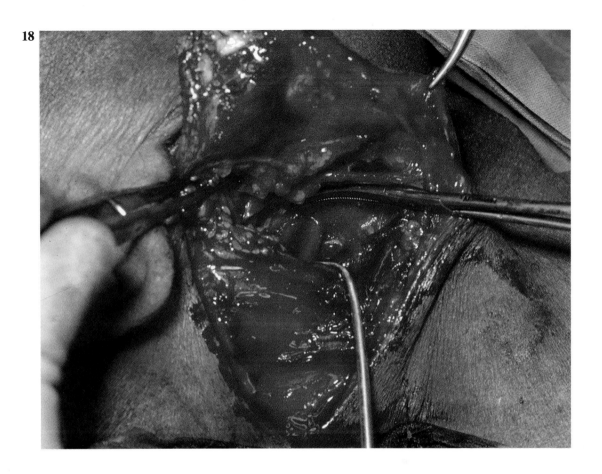

18 Exposure of stylohyoid muscle. The dissection of the previous illustration has now been further deepened to expose the stylohyoid muscle. The retractor holds down the anterior border of the sterno-mastoid muscle and also points at the posterior belly of the digastric muscle while the curved artery forceps now points to the stylohyoid muscle. In the orientation of these illustrations, the two deeper muscles,

the digastric and the stylohyoid, appear to be running almost directly upwards and also away from the observer.

Once these muscles have been clearly identified it is time to make the facial part of the incision. Above the stylohyoid muscle, the white object at the very tip of the curved artery forceps is the external carotid artery, seen just before it plunges into the deep part of the parotid salivary gland.

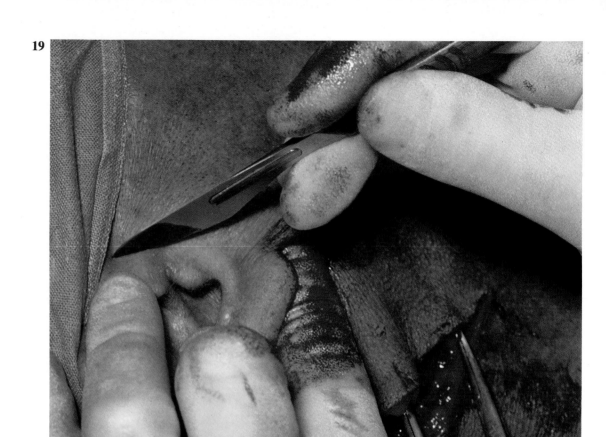

19 **The facial part of the cervico-mastoid-facial incision is now made,** starting from the zygoma above and running downwards along the skin crease in front of the pinna to meet the upper end of the mastoid incision. Note the surgeon's left forefinger pushing the lump away from the line of the incision.

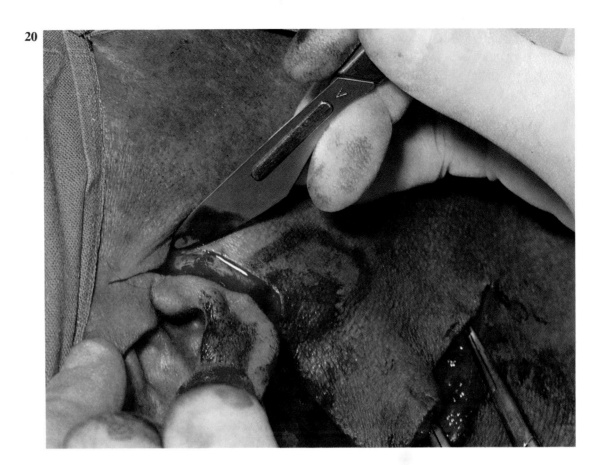

20 The facial incision is cautiously deepened with the knife, still making sure that there is no question of cutting into the lump. The deepening is for only 2 mm or 3 mm, when the surgeon will find evidence that his knife blade is reaching a very fine natural plane of cleavage between the cartilage of the external auditory meatus posteriorly and the parotid gland anteriorly.

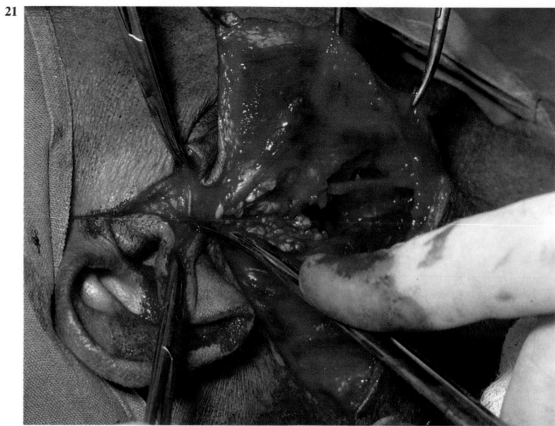

21 Extending the plane downwards. At the lower end of the facial incision, a few touches with curved scissors extend the zone of this plane of cleavage downwards towards the neck. Note how the anterior skin-flap is being elevated to pull the lump forwards, so that it is not encroached upon by the cuts of the scissors.

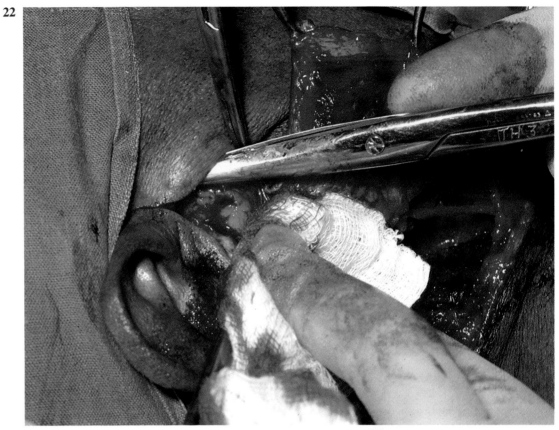

22 Development of cleavage with artery forceps. The plane of cleavage
in front of the cartilage of the external auditory meatus is developed by
blunt dissection with artery forceps. In this illustration the pair of scissors
is only being used to demonstrate how deeply the dissection has already
proceeded.

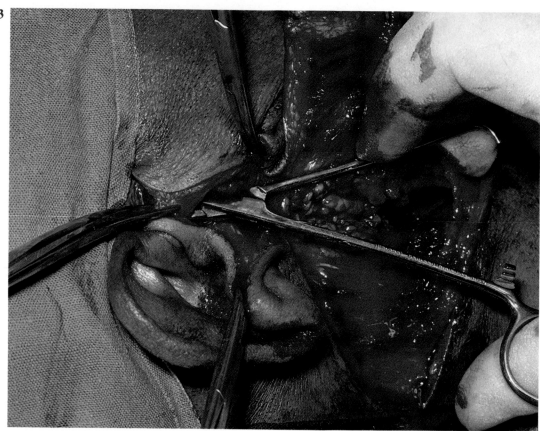

23 **Blunt and sharp dissection.** While there are some blood vessels in the connective tissue occupying this plane, much of the tissue is avascular. This illustration shows the technique of combining blunt with sharp dissection to deepen the plane. The pair of artery forceps has been pushed into the tissue so that its points project beyond a bridge of tissue, and the bridge is being cut with a pair of curved scissors. For right-handed operators, it is convenient to be able to cut with the left hand.

The artery forceps blades protect deeper structures from injury. This procedure is perfectly safe in the region of the plane lying immediately anterior to the cartilage of the external auditory meatus.

24 Use of artery forceps. The artery forceps is opening up the plane yet more deeply. This is a beautiful surgical plane, very easily opened with a minimum of bleeding in a case, like this, in which the patient has not had a previous operation upon the parotid. Of course, if there has been a previous operation, or if the parotidectomy is being done for generalised inflammatory disease, the plane may be much more difficult to dissect open. In any case, it is necessary to persist with the deepening of this plane between the cartilage of the external meatus posteriorly and the parotid salivary gland anteriorly until with one's finger tips one feels bone of the external auditory meatus. As soon as bone can be felt, it is vital that the dissection should not further be deepened at this stage, because the territory of the facial nerve is now being approached.

At this point the author usually reduces the strength of his diathermy apparatus to the minimal power in the cutting mode (the author always uses cutting diathermy for coagulating bleeding points because the zone of tissue destruction around the diathermy point is smaller with the cutting than with the coagulating current).

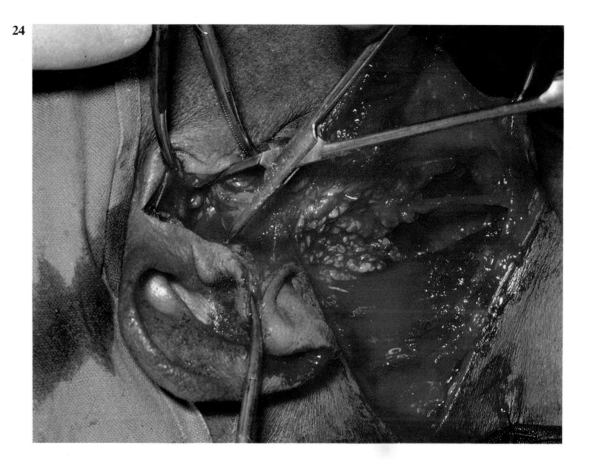
24

25 Finding facial nerve trunk. This is the
most important of all illustrations seen so far.
It contains the key to finding the trunk of the
facial nerve.

In the neck, the two retractors are holding
open the space between the anterior borders of
three muscles (the sternomastoid, posterior
belly of the digastric and stylohyoid) and the
posterior or lower pole of the parotid salivary
gland. In the face, the surgeon is demonstrating with a pair of dissecting forceps the
space in front of the cartilage of the external
auditory meatus, the latter becoming the
bony external auditory meatus in the depth
of the dissection. Between these two cavities,
and clearly seen in this illustration is a bridge
of tissue about 4 cm wide, and it is the whittling away of this bridge of tissues in small
portions at a time that ultimately leads the
surgeon to the trunk of the facial nerve.

Incidentally, the author does not recom-
mend using retractors to hold the parotid
gland out of the way. The anterior of the pair
of retractors in this illustration was used very
gently for a few seconds only, but normally
the operator uses only his finger gently to
push the gland forwards. Injudicious pressure from a retractor can burst a parotid
tumour even though there has been no direct
breach of its capsule.

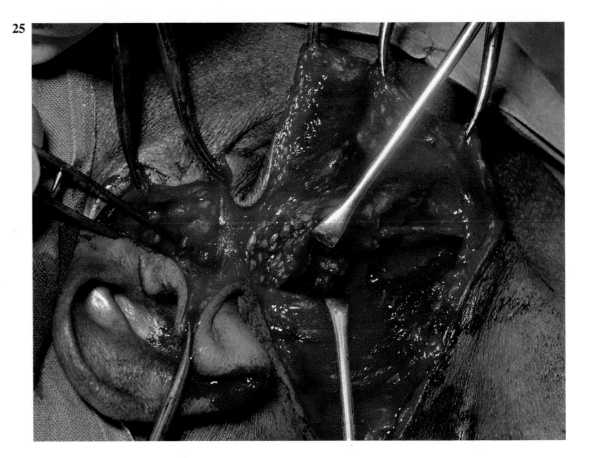

25

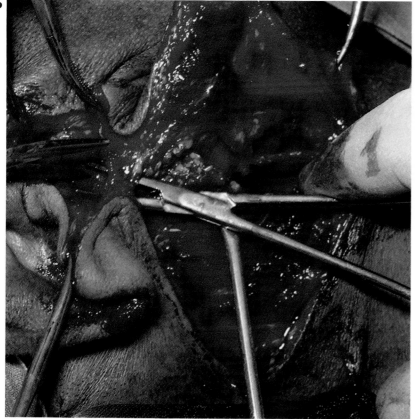 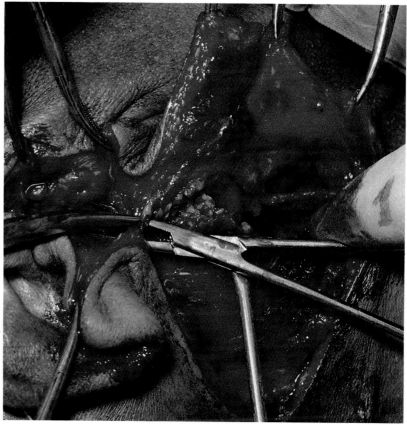

26 and 27   Method of cutting through the bridge of tissues so as to expose the facial nerve. A pair of artery forceps is pushed through the bridge so as to isolate from below a portion of tissue about 2 mm or 3 mm deep, the point of the instrument emerging at the upper border of the band. The separated tissue is carefully wiped free of blood and inspected to make sure that it contains no important structures, and then divided with scissors. Should there be a vessel somewhere in the portion of tissue, the rest of the portion is divided and then the vessel controlled with diathermy (having removed the metal artery forceps first!) before it is divided. No division of tissue takes place without the artery forceps in position to protect the deeper tissues, and every precaution is taken to avoid cutting any formed structure in the separated segment of the bridge. This process is repeated many times over; gradually the bridge of tissues is destroyed.

28 A good view of the nerve. At last! The moment the surgeon has been eagerly awaiting. When the artery forceps was inserted on the previous occasion, on separating the blades the facial nerve trunk and (on this occasion) its bifurcation into the main upper and lower subdivisions were seen. The surgeon's forefinger is pushing the parotid salivary gland forwards to give a good view of the nerve, and an artery forceps has been inserted under the nerve to bring it forwards and make it more easily visible. In this particular patient it was known that the tumour was in the deep part of the gland and therefore that the deep aspect of the facial nerve would need to be mobilised to remove the deep part of the gland. However, in the normal way, at this stage of the operation one does not necessarily know whether a lump is superficial or deep to the nerve, and therefore it is quite likely that it will not be necessary to dissect the deep aspect of the facial nerve off the deep portion of the parotid. In these circumstances it would be quite wrong to elevate the nerve in this way for the purposes of photography, because dissection of the deep aspect further destroys the blood supply of the facial nerve and must make it more vulnerable to trauma and thus make more likely a temporary paralysis of the facial muscles.

Even though the rest of the course of the facial nerve and its branches may be grossly distorted by the presence of a large tumour, in the author's experience the trunk of the nerve is always to be found by following this set procedure. The surgeon should, however, be on the alert for the possibility that there has been an early division of the trunk

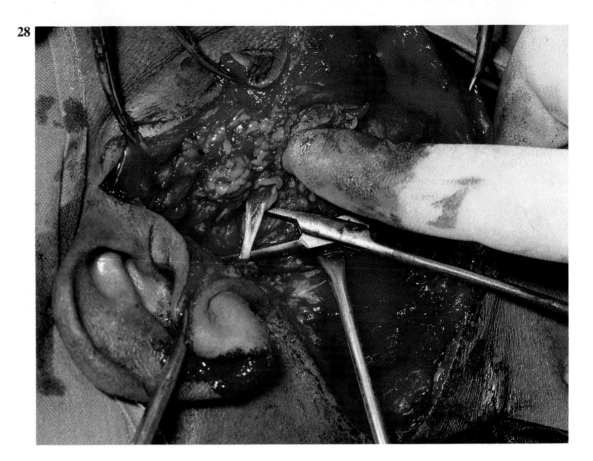

28

within the facial canal, resulting in not one facial nerve trunk but apparently two! It is theoretically possible that one might find one of these trunks and then become careless and destroy the other during the subsequent dissection. This calamity can be avoided by making sure that one has found a bifurcation as well as a main trunk.

29 Dissection of uppermost and lowermost branches. The surgeon's objective now is to dissect the uppermost branch of the upper division and the lowermost branch of the lower division right forwards to the margin of the skin incision. These manoeuvres set the limits of the dissection above and below and form a framework within which dissection of the other branches of the facial nerve forwards from the bifurcation result in the separation of the superficial part of the parotid salivary gland.

In theory it does not matter whether the uppermost branch of the upper division or the lowermost branch of the lower division is tackled first. In practice, it is easier to deal with whichever branch is furthest from the tumour. Clearly the lowermost branch of the lower division was in this case travelling close to the tumour; therefore it was decided to dissect first the uppermost branch of the upper division.

The illustration shows the commencement of the dissection. The blades of the artery forceps are slightly parted and show between them the trunk of the facial nerve just proximal to its bifurcation. The artery forceps are about to be plunged into the tissues immediately superficial to the upper division of the nerve. The surgeon must take a view as to exactly which direction the nerve is taking once it has disappeared from view into the as yet undissected tissue; with experience he will find the decision more easily and more accurately made. Certainly the uppermost branch of the upper division nearly always runs directly vertically upwards, parallel with the cartilage of the external auditory meatus and at a distance of about 1.5 cm in front of it.

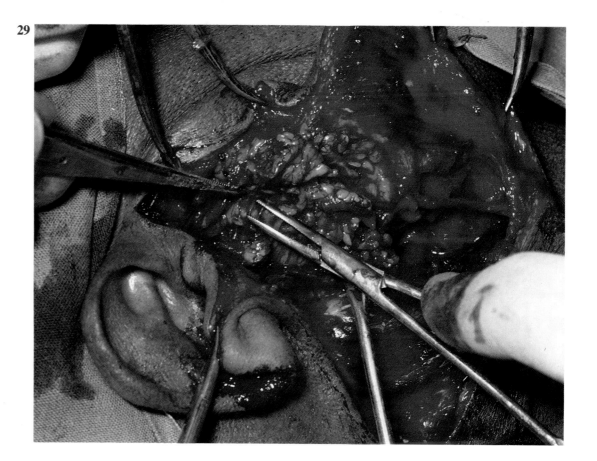

29

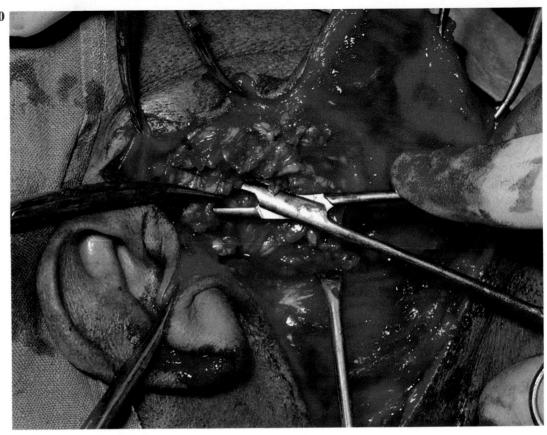

30 Artery forceps in tissue. The artery forceps has now been plunged into the tissue immediately beyond and superficial to the commencement of the upper division of the facial nerve; the scissors are cutting between the blades of the forceps in the usual manner.

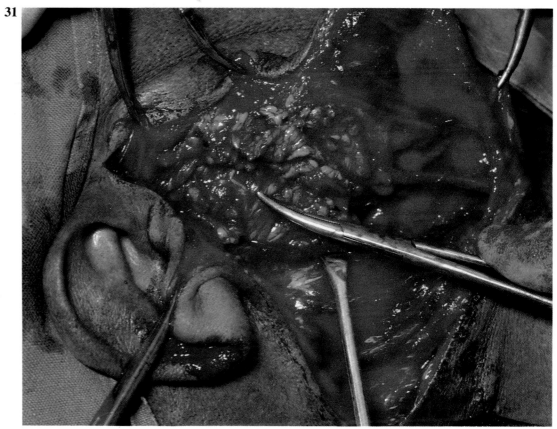

31 **The bridge of tissues between the jaws of the artery forceps of 30 has now been divided to expose another 0.5 cm (5 mm) of the uppermost branch of the upper division.** The artery forceps overlies the lowermost branch of the lower division and points towards the uppermost branch of the upper division. Those with keen eyesight may see the beginning of a forward running branch of the upper main division, just where the latter is plunging into undissected tissues.

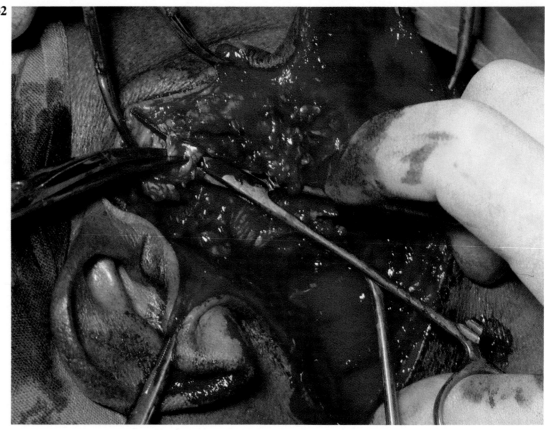

32 and 33 Further stages of dissection of the uppermost branch of the upper division, i.e. the temporal branch. In **32** another tissue bridge is being divided superficial to this nerve branch: **33** shows the complete dissection of this branch right up to the skin margin in the region of the highest of the artery forceps on the anterior skin margin. Also clearly visible in this illustration are the zygomatic and the upper buccal branch which are coming off the anterior margin of the main upper subdivision of the facial nerve. This view is also useful to show the general position of the tumour, which lies deep to the tissue below the main trunk and the lower main subdivision of the facial nerve.

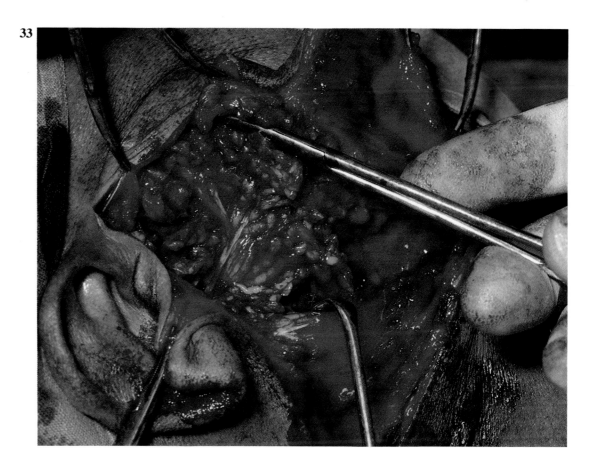

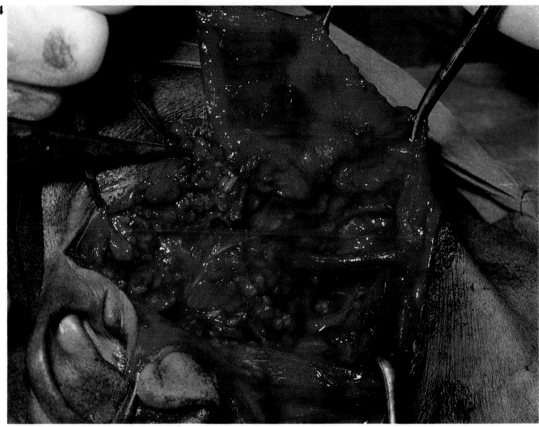

34 **Exposure of platysmal branch.** The surgeon then uses exactly the same process to expose the lowermost branch of the lower division, i.e. the platysmal branch. To save unnecessary repetition, **34** shows this branch completely dissected right up to the skin margin, in this view not far behind the artery forceps to the right of the picture, and in front of the common facial vein. Not far anterior to the bifurcation, two branches (probably buccal) are visible running forwards from the lower main sub-division.

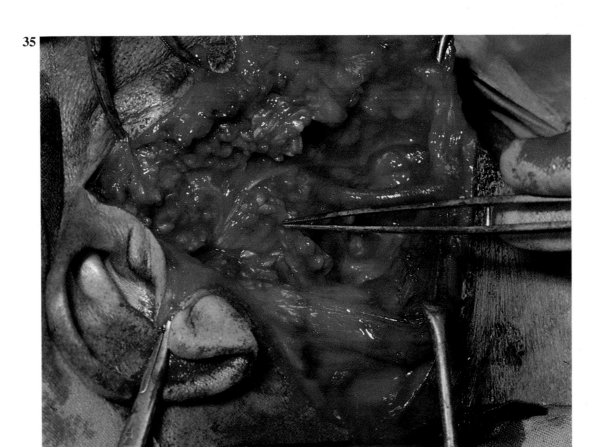

35 The dissecting forceps lie on the surface of the tumour, although the latter is still covered with some normal parotid tissue. The superficial part of the parotid salivary gland is clearly visible in front of the main branches of the nerve as they fan upwards and downwards. In removing the deep part of the parotid gland, it would be easy to injure the peripheral branches of the facial nerve from their deep aspects. It is therefore imperative to dissect the branches far enough forwards so that they can be under continuous view during the rest of the dissection. To do this the superficial part of the parotid has to be completely mobilised and it is probably therefore better removed.

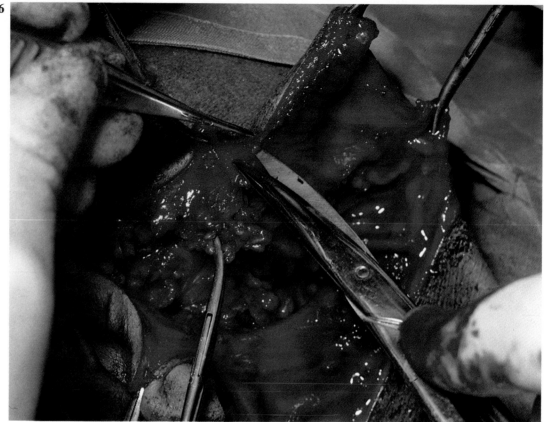

36   Elevation of anterior skin-flap. The anterior skin-flap is now being elevated using a pair of scissors, backwards traction on the superficial parotid being provided with the aid of the artery forceps shown. The anterior skin-flap should not be raised until the position of the lump in relation to the facial nerve is clearly known. The author has seen the facial nerve divided during the raising of the skin-flap because a tumour in the deep part of the gland had pushed the nerve and its branches outwards so strongly that the superficial part of the parotid had atrophied and the nerves were lying in the subcutaneous plane. The reflection of the skin-flap should proceed forward until the anterior margin of the parotid salivary gland is reached, about halfway forwards along the masseter muscle.

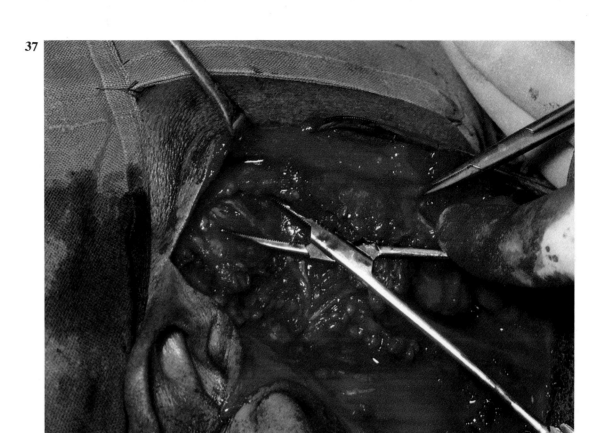

37 The beginning of the dissection forwards of the superficial part of the parotid. The zygomatic branch to the eye is being traced forwards in the usual way.

38 Completion of dissection of upper half of superficial parotid. At this stage the dissection of the upper half of the superficial parotid has been completed and the upper division of the facial nerve is now completely exposed. Note how the temporal branch gives off the zygomatic branches and there are two upper buccal branches, one arising at an early stage from the main upper subdivision of the nerve and the other arising from the temporal branch at the same point as the zygomatic branches arise. The yellow lobulated tissue of the superficial parotid is clearly visible between the buccal branches and the gauze swab, the latter being used to stanch by pressure from a finger tip a bleeding point that was proving awkward to secure.

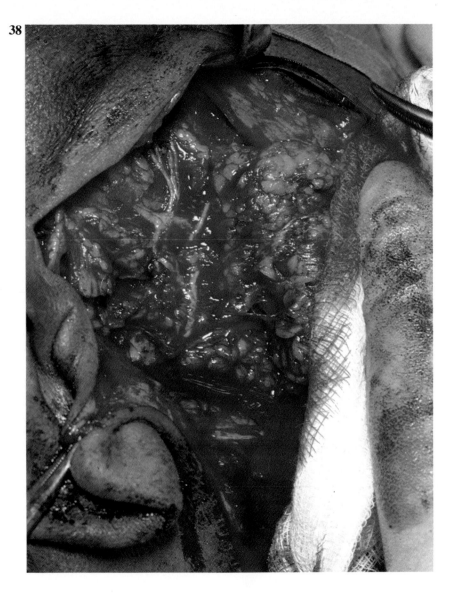

38

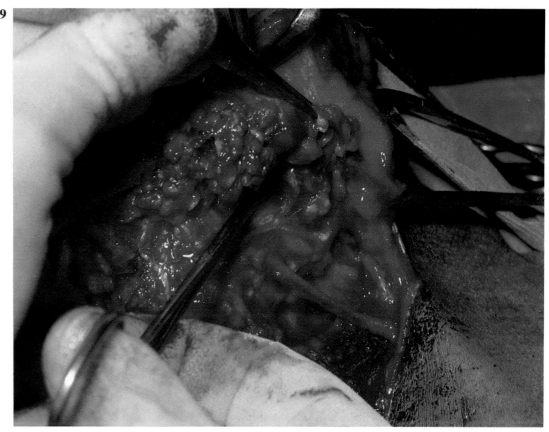

39 Lower half of the superficial parotid being dissected forwards by dissection of the mandibular branch of the facial nerve forward from its point of origin from the lower main subdivision. The dissecting forceps are being used to pick up tissue immediately superficial to and beyond where the nerve to the angle of the mouth has so far been exposed.

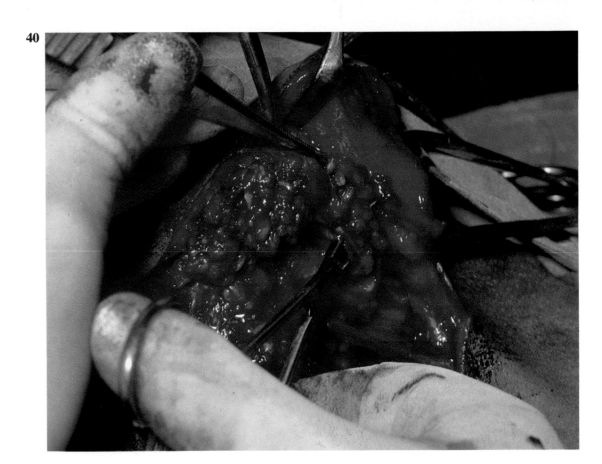

40   The mandibular nerve to the angle of the mouth is being demonstrated by the artery forceps immediately deep to it. The dissection has to continue in a line running forwards to the point which the surgeon is demonstrating with the tip of his dissecting forceps near the top of the picture. At that stage the nerve will have passed the anterior margin of the parotid salivary gland and will no longer be at risk during removal of the gland.

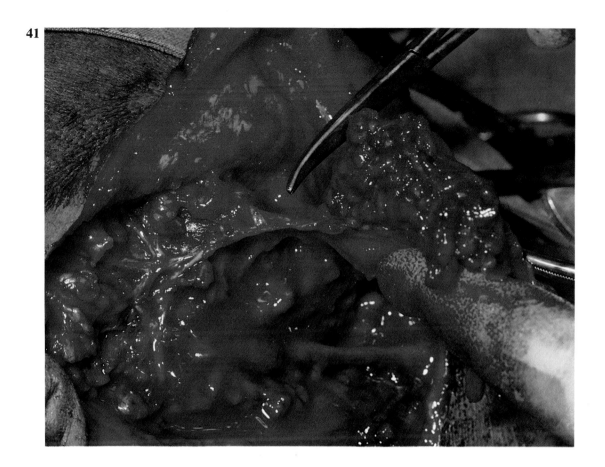

41 **The superficial part of the parotid has now been almost completely dissected off the facial nerve branches and the deep portion of the gland.** One shred of tissue remains at the region where the parotid duct joins the superficial part of the gland, and division of this piece of tissue will result in the gland superficially being free apart from the parotid duct itself. The artery forceps is pointing at the parotid duct. Finding the duct is easier if one remembers that it runs horizontally and opens into the mouth at the level of the second upper molar tooth.

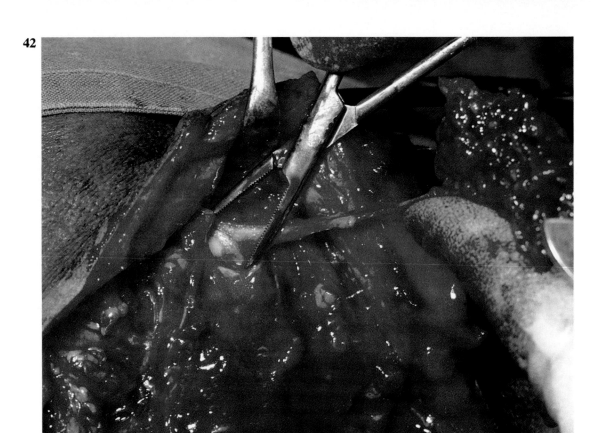

42 Dissection of parotid duct. The remaining strand of tissue linking the superficial with the deep portion of the parotid has now been divided and the parotid duct dissected well forwards until the fat of the buccinator fat pad becomes visible. Although the author cannot prove this statement, he feels that it is important to take the main parotid duct as far forwards as shown to ensure that the duct draining the deep lobe, which enters the main duct well forward along the masseter muscle, is destroyed. While it is not relevant in this particular patient because the deep lobe is going to be removed, in other patients in whom the deep lobe is not to be removed, it is important that its drainage should be destroyed so that it atrophies and cannot give rise to a parotid fistula.

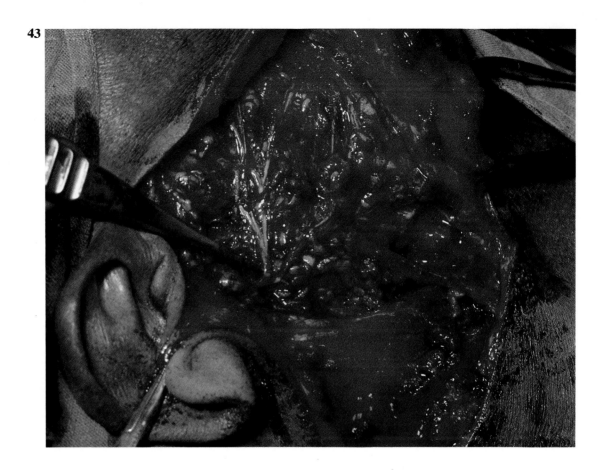

43 The superficial part of the parotid has been removed and the trunk, bifurcation and branches of the facial nerve are clearly displayed throughout their parotid course. The lump lies in the part of the parotid deep to the nerve, and dissecting forceps are used to show that the trunk and bifurcation of the nerve have already been dissected free of the underlying deep parotid (see **28**). The lobulated tissue of the deep part of the parotid is clearly visible deep to the facial nerve and its branches.

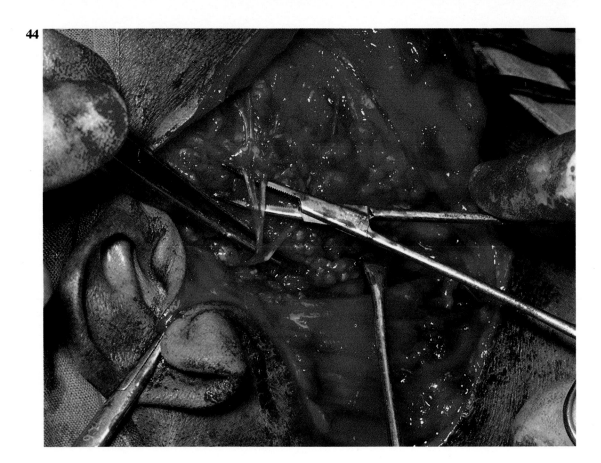

44   Freeing of facial nerve and branches. The process of freeing the facial nerve and its branches from the deep part of the parotid salivary gland is being continued; in this illustration the upper division and its main branches are being freed by dissection with an artery forceps deep to the nerve. Slight tension to aid the dissection is being maintained with the dissecting forceps in the surgeon's left hand, but it is very important that no excess tension should be used, because the facial nerve takes a long time to recover from the effects of stretching.

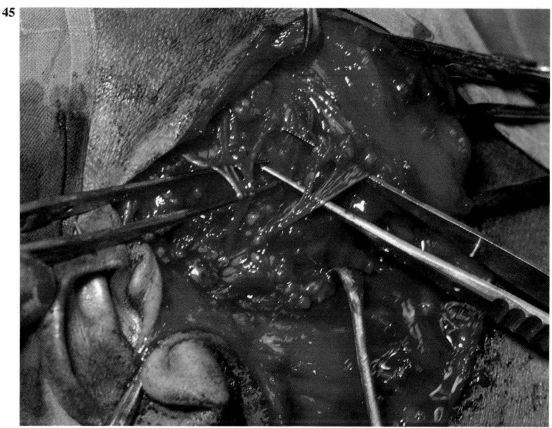

45 Separation of facial nerve from parotid gland. The process of separating the facial nerve branches from the underlying deep parotid gland has now continued to include the inferior main subdivision of the nerve and its major branches. The facial nerve trunk and all its branches have now been elevated off the surface of the deep part of the parotid. The way has thus been prepared for mobilisation of the deep part with its enclosed tumour.

46   The key to the mobilisation of the deep part of the parotid is the fact that the external carotid artery enters the inferior pole of the deep part, traverses the deep part to the upper pole, and there emerges either as the external carotid artery or (if it has divided a little earlier) as the superficial temporal artery running upwards to the forehead and the maxillary artery running forwards deep to the mandibular ramus. Any attempt to remove the deep lobe without first securing the major arteries would entail an extreme hazard from blood loss. Because bleeding from the external carotid artery if it is cut is even more severe than from the superficial temporal and maxillary arteries, it is usually wise to secure the external carotid artery first, but if the lump overlies the external carotid it might be wiser to start the mobilisation from the top of the deep part of the gland by finding and dividing between ligatures the superficial temporal and maxillary arteries. In the present case, there was no contraindication to the more usual attack on the external carotid artery first.

This illustration shows how the artery is found. The retractor is holding downwards the anterior border of the sternomastoid, that is the upper border of the muscle as this picture is orientated. Below the blade of the retractor can be seen the bright red of the posterior belly of the digastric muscle. The dissecting forceps lies with its tips under the external carotid artery as it rises from the neck deep to the darker stylohyoid muscle, and the artery forceps lies deep to the artery just as it is about to plunge into the parotid salivary gland. If the artery is found at the upper border of stylohyoid muscle in this way, it is virtually impossible that the internal carotid artery might be mistaken for the external carotid artery. However, it is always a wise precaution to make sure that the artery one is going to tie has at least one branch arising from it, because the internal carotid artery gives off no branches in the neck.

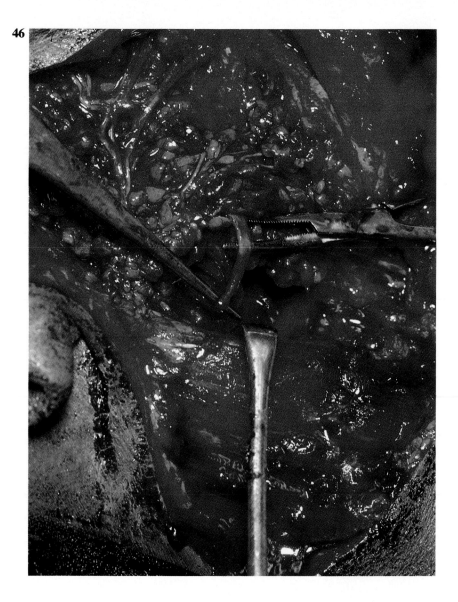

46

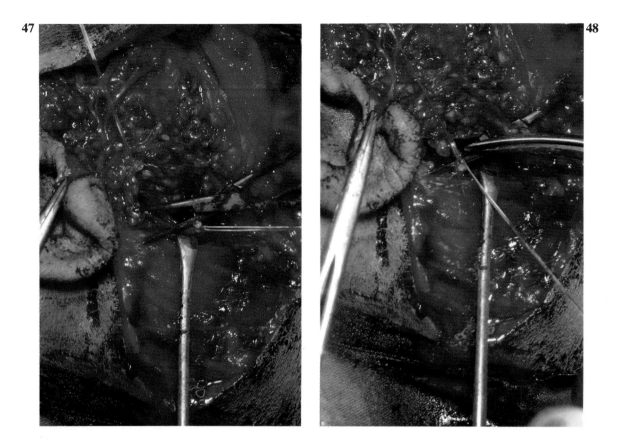

47 Aneurysm needles have been used to pass ligatures around the external carotid artery and it has been tied before division. The author always puts two ligatures on the proximal (cervical) end for safety.

48 Companion vein to external carotid artery. Sometimes there is a considerable companion vein to the external carotid artery; this illustration shows the vein after tying and just about to be divided.

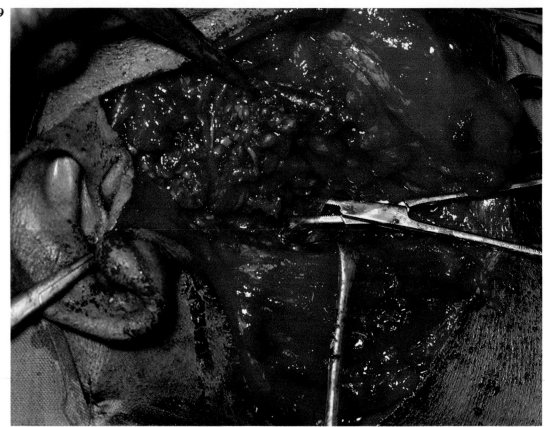

49 Mobilisation of the nerves superficial to the gland is now continued using the usual combination of blunt and sharp dissection. The artery forceps in this illustration is lying beneath the stylomandibular ligament, a band of fascia attached to the styloid process posteriorly and the angle of the mandible anteriorly. This ligament often produces a waist-like constriction in a tumour of the deep lobe, and the division of this ligament greatly increases the mobility of the lower pole of the deep portion of gland. Note how the mobilisation of the branches of the facial nerve has allowed them to be pushed upwards, while the lower pole of the gland is delivered from the lateral pharyngeal recess.

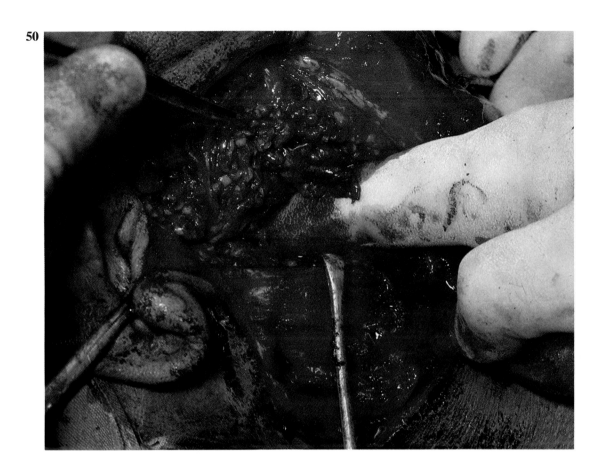

50 Freeing of deep part of the gland. The surgeon's finger is demonstrating how completely the lower pole of the deep part of the gland has been freed. It is not possible to proceed any further from the inferior direction under vision and therefore attention must be directed elsewhere. Again, note how all the branches of the facial nerve have been pushed upwards to allow delivery of the lower pole of the gland from its bed.

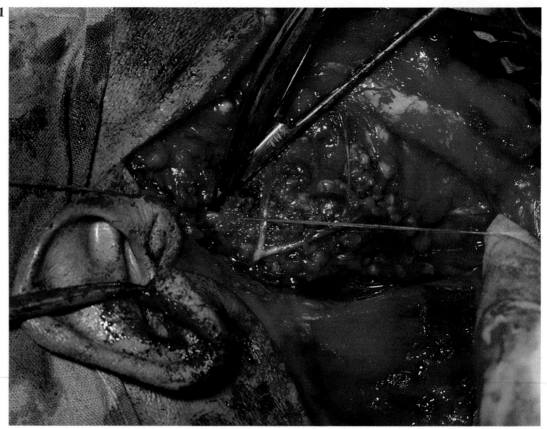

51 Dissection near the upper border of the parotid salivary gland in the region of the zygoma leads to the identification of the upper end of the external carotid artery or (if the latter has divided at an earlier stage) the superficial temporal artery. Ligatures have been placed around the vessel in two places and it is to be divided. This step is an important one for achieving the mobilisation of the upper pole of the deep part of the parotid.

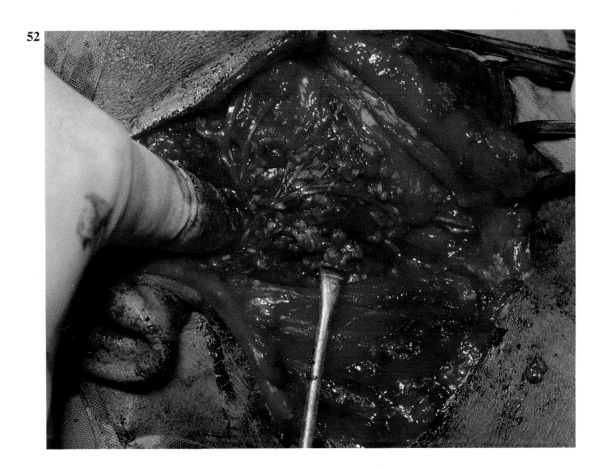

52 Mobilisation of the upper pole of the gland permits a certain degree of displacement of the whole gland downwards behind the branches of the facial nerve.

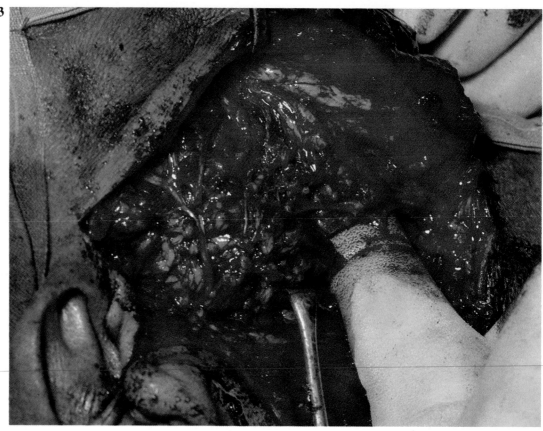

53 Adhesions of connective tissues. The surgeon's exploring forefinger demonstrates that there are still adhesions of connective tissue anchoring the anterior border of the deep pole of the gland to the back and deep surface of the ramus of the mandible. Some of these adhesions can be broken down by blunt dissection with the finger, because the blood vessels in this region are small and unlikely to bleed dangerously, but such blunt dissection is only safe provided that the surgeon is quite certain that he is not anywhere near the region of the tumour.

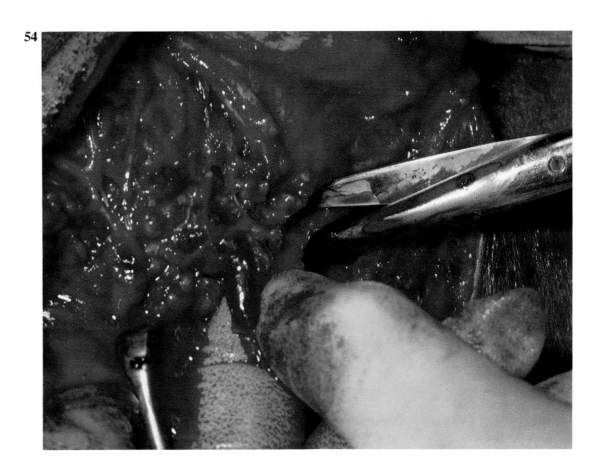

54 Division of tissue. As the mobilisation of the anterior border of the gland is continued, it becomes increasingly easy to pull down the tissue attaching the anterior part of the parotid to the jaw and to divide it with scissors under direct vision.

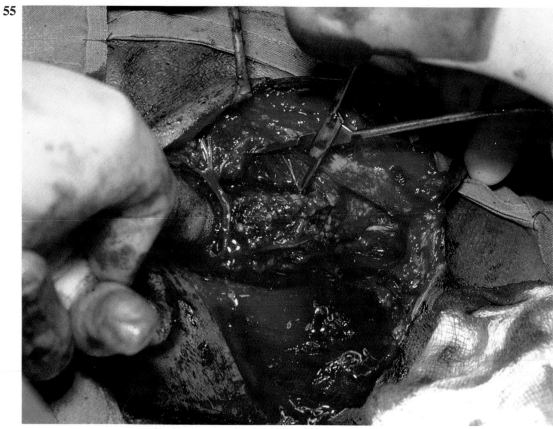

55 Detachment of parotid from ramus. A few touches with an artery forceps are sufficient to complete the detachment of the anterior border of the deep part of the parotid from the back of the ramus of the mandible. This illustration also shows how the surgeon's left index finger is pushing down the deep part of the parotid behind the facial nerve and its branches, so that the lower pole is being dislocated downwards to overlap the anterior border of the sternomastoid muscle in the lower part of the dissection.

56 Dissection is now carried out in front of the point where the superficial temporal artery was tied in order to find and divide between ligatures the maxillary artery. It is particularly important to secure control of this vessel before it is divided, because the distal cut end retracts behind the mandible and zygoma and it becomes a severe technical problem to gain control of the bleeding. Should this accident occur, several deep sutures should be inserted into the fossa which is bleeding, because this is usually the best way of controlling the bleeding.

Note in this illustration that ligatures have been placed round a branch of the external carotid artery, probably the lingual artery, which was getting in the way of the freeing of the anterior border of the parotid. It is unusual to meet a large vessel in this region but the deep part of this particular parotid salivary gland extended further forwards than usual.

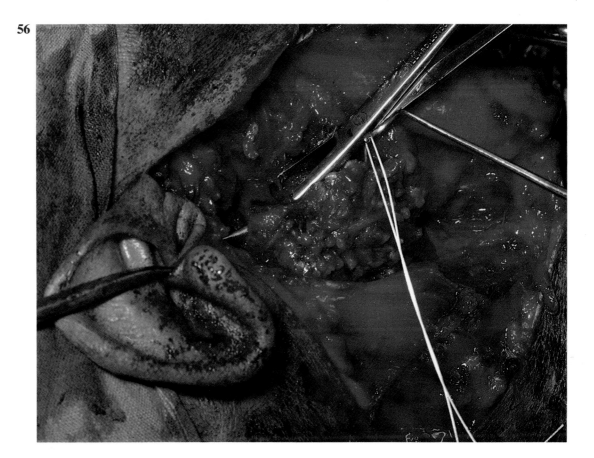

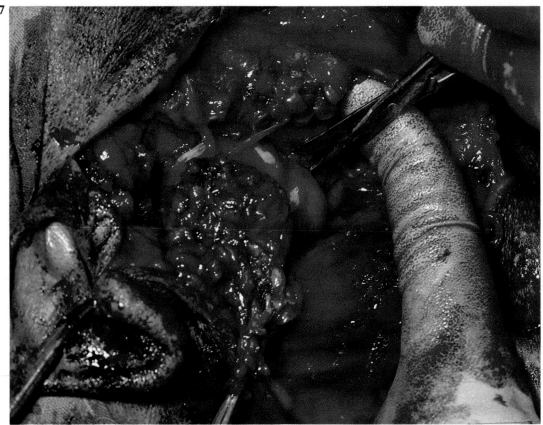

57 The deep part of the parotid has now been almost completely dislocated from its bed and delivered below the mobilised branches of the facial nerve. However, a few shreds of diaphanous connective tissue are still attaching the deep aspect of the tumour in the depth of the gland to the region of the lateral pharyngeal wall. The surgeon's left index finger is displacing the pharyngeal wall and the pterygoid muscles forward so that under direct vision these strands of tissue can be divided.

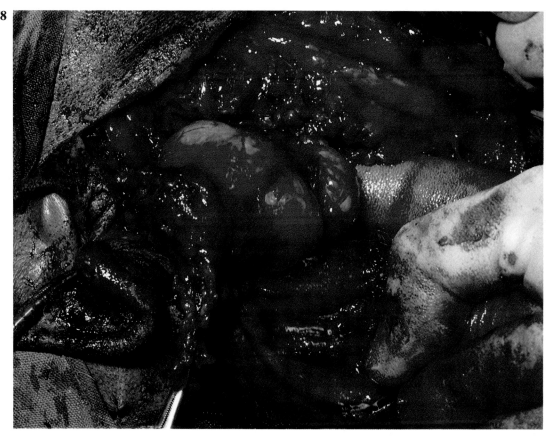

58 The surgeon's right index finger is now testing whether the deep portion of the parotid with its enclosed tumour is free from the lateral pharyngeal wall. This illustration well shows the main portion of the remaining parotid, then deep to that the pale-yellow surface of the tumour shining through the covering of connective tissue that the surgeon has been at pains to preserve over the surface of the tumour. Note particularly the deep lobulation of the inferior pole of the tumour, so that it looks in this view almost as though they are two separate tumours. The stylomandibular ligament occupied and presumably produced this deep groove.

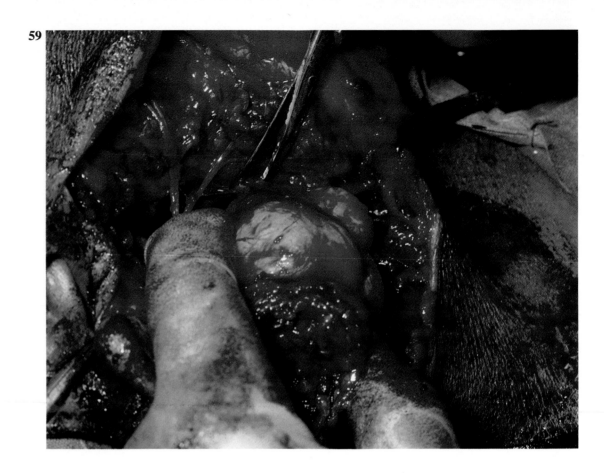

59 Dividing strands of fibrous tissue. The last few touches to divide the remaining strands of fibrous tissue, and then the deep part of the parotid and the lobulated tumour will be completely mobilised. Note how the tissue deep to the nerve has been delivered from beneath the lower border of the facial nerve system, the nerves having been pushed upwards after being well mobilised.

60 Lobulated tumour in deep lobe excised.
The deep lobe with its attached lobulated yellow tumour is now completely free and its bed deep to the trunk and branches of the facial nerve is clearly exposed. Note the sternomastoid and posterior belly of the digastric muscles in this view, but the stylohyoid is not so clearly visible. The tumour is very much larger than would have been suspected by examination from the outside, and having expanded to fill nearly all the space available to it in the lateral pharyngeal recess there is little normal tissue surrounding it for the surgeon to preserve. However, what little there was has been preserved and nowhere is the surface of the tumour laid bare. Thus the object of the operation, to remove the lump in the parotid salivary gland with a margin of normal tissue and with preservation of the facial nerve if possible, has been achieved.

Details of closure will be shown in connection with another operation (see **87** and **88**).

60

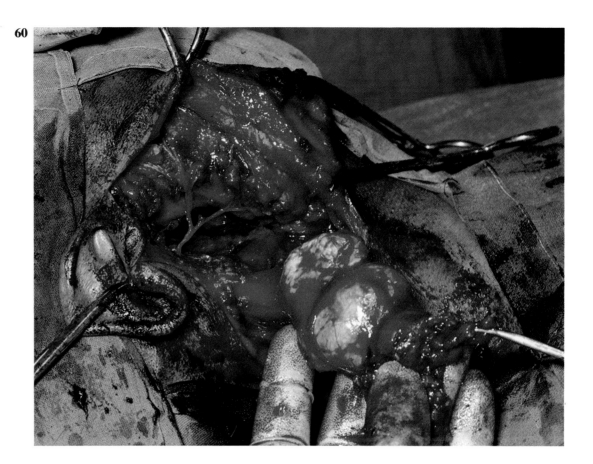

Superficial parotidectomy with a variation in technique

The next set of illustrations (**61** to **88**) show a different parotidectomy operation. The differences include the fact that the lesion is on the left instead of the right, that only a superficial parotidectomy was needed rather than a total parotidectomy, that certain details of the arrangement of the anaesthetic and the patient's position are emphasised here, having escaped notice in the first operation, and most important of all, that the method of tracing forward the branches of the facial nerve, starting with the uppermost part of the upper division and the lowermost branch of the lower division, was modified to suit the circumstances of this particular lump. The lump in question was so closely overhanging and adjacent to the upper division of the facial nerve that any attempt to dissect forwards along the upper division of the nerve would have been hazardous,

because it would probably have ended up with breaching the capsule of the tumour. Therefore, the alternative strategy of dissecting the branches of the facial nerve from below upwards was adopted. Once the lower part of the lump could be lifted off the lower branches of the facial nerve, it became easier to separate the lump and surrounding tissues from the upper branches of the nerve.

The same principle can be applied in the reverse way for a lump in the lower portion of the gland; the branches of the nerves are dissected in order from above downwards. Such variations emphasise the point that no two operations for parotidectomy are completely alike; the surgeon must be prepared to deal with the situation as he finds it.

61 Position of the patient on the operating table. Note particularly how the arm is well wrapped around to prevent contact of the bare flesh with the metal of the operating table which might lead to diathermy burns, that the heels are supported on a soft cushion to reduce the risk of deep-vein thrombosis in the calf, and that the head is only turned slightly to the right (see description in **17** for the explanation why it is important not to turn the head too far to the opposite side). The position of the head is maintained with the aid of the head ring on which it lies.

Electrocardiograph leads have been applied because the anaesthetist was going to induce severe hypotension with intravenous sodium nitro-

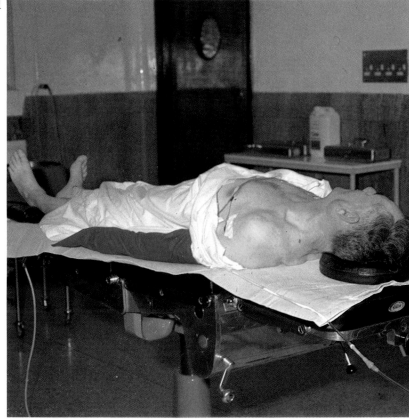

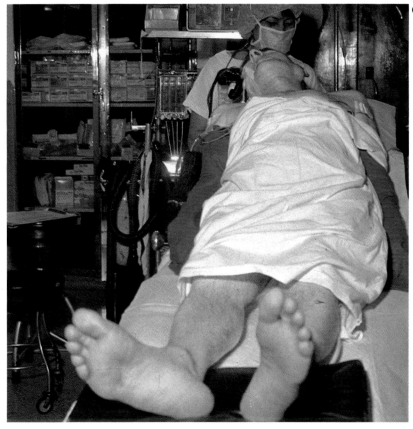

prusside. Blood pressure was accordingly being monitored with an intra-arterial line. The arrangement of the anaesthetic tubing and of the rubber tube leading from the ordinary sphygmomanometer is also shown. There is a head-up tilt on the operating table although this might not be obvious in this illustration. In any case, the tilt is not sufficient because the bulge of the external jugular and posterior facial veins can be clearly seen in the neck. Venous oozing from the operation field can be considerably reduced if sufficient tilt is achieved to cause the external jugular vein to collapse.

62 Another general view of the operating table. It emphasises the tucking in of the arms, the protection of the calves, the turning of the head to the opposite side, and the head-up tilt. It also shows how the anaesthetist and apparatus are concentrated in a prolongation of the head-end of the operating table. The space at each side of the operating table and in a similar area beyond the head-end of the operating table is free for the surgeon and his two assistants.

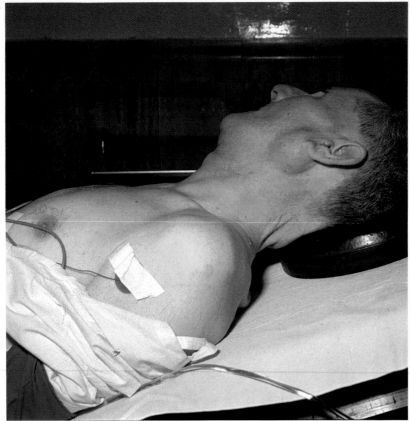

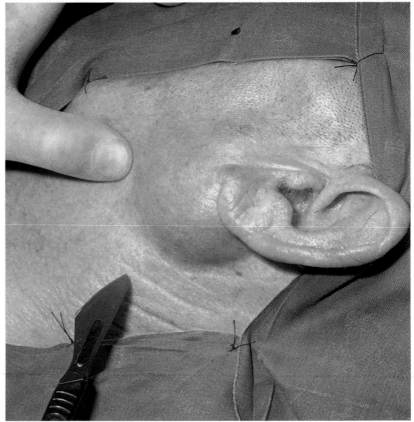

63   Close up of the operative area and immediate surroundings shows the taping of the left eye and also the fact that the external jugular vein is now collapsed. The sternomastoid muscle is bulging but there is no sign of the vein running across it towards the lower border of the lump. Notice how the upper margin of the lump extends almost to the zygoma, the bulge of which is clearly visible. The details of the shaving of the head around the ear and neck are also obvious.

64   Cervical incision. The surgeon's left thumb is on the angle of the jaw and the point of the blade of the scalpel indicates the upper skin crease of the neck in which the cervical part of the incision will be made. Note again how far below the angle of the jaw is the cervical incision.

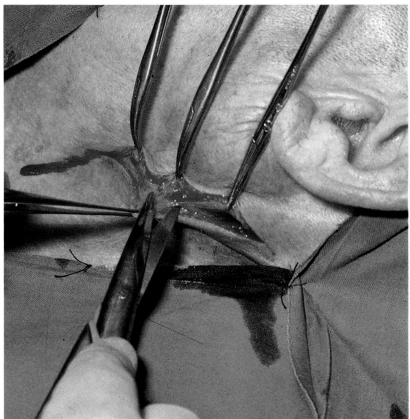

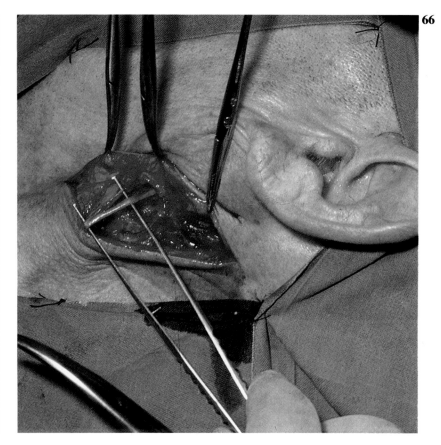

65 The cervical incision has been made. Three pairs of artery forceps have been applied to the subcutaneous tissue of the upper aspect of the incision and are holding up that skin-flap. The dissection has been deepened through platysma, along the lower skin-flap rather than the upper, to avoid getting too near the lump.

66 The great auricular nerve has been demonstrated and a segment of it is about to be cut out.

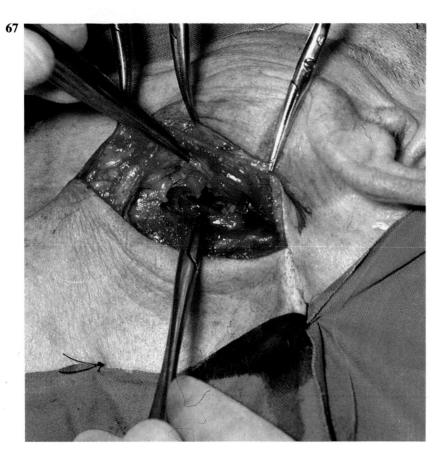

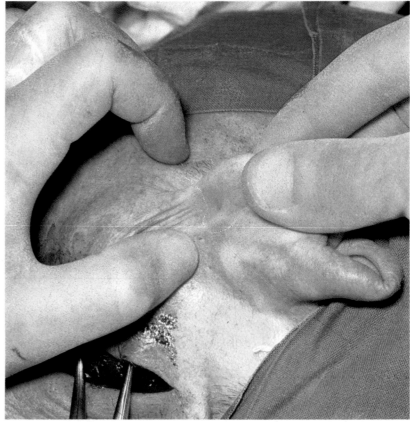

67   Cervical incision deepened to expose three important muscular landmarks. The artery forceps in the surgeon's right hand is hooked over the anterior border of the sternomastoid muscle and its tips are resting on the posterior belly of the digastric. On an even deeper plane, the paler fibres of the stylohyoid muscle can be seen as well.

68   Surgeon preparing to make the mastoid part of the cervico-mastoid-facial incision. His left index finger and thumb are gently pulling the lump forwards away from the pinna, while the right hand is pulling the pinna backwards. Having established the best point at which to make the incision, the surgeon will ask his assistant to take over the hold on the pinna, so that the surgeon's right hand is now free to make the incision. Carelessness at this stage can result in the knife cutting into the tumour and a spillage of neoplastic cells.

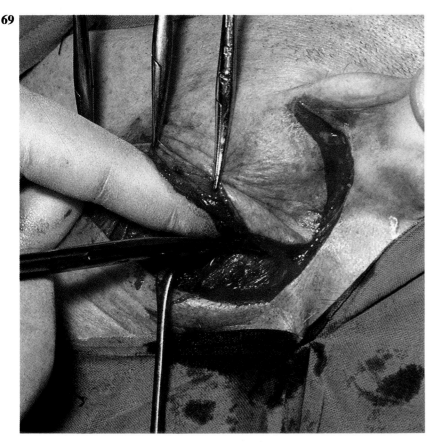

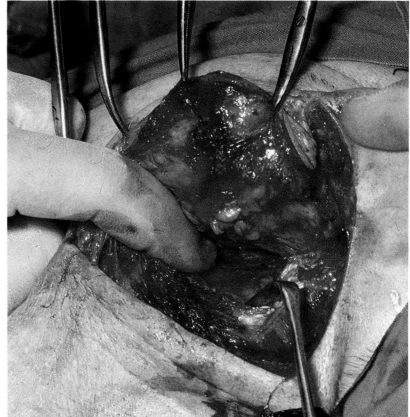

69 **The mastoid part of the incision has now been made**, and the surgeon's left index finger is pushing the lump forwards, away from the pair of scissors with which he is following the anterior border of the sternomastoid towards the mastoid process.

70 **The making of the mastoid part of the incision has made it easier to dissect the posterior belly of the digastric and the stylohyoid muscles upwards along their anterior borders.** In this illustration the retractor is hooked round the anterior border of the sternomastoid muscle, while the left index finger rests on the anterior border of the posterior belly of the digastric and, deep to that, on the stylohyoid muscle. The lump is within the upper portion of the wound but is covered by parotid tissue so that though bulging its surface is not actually visible.

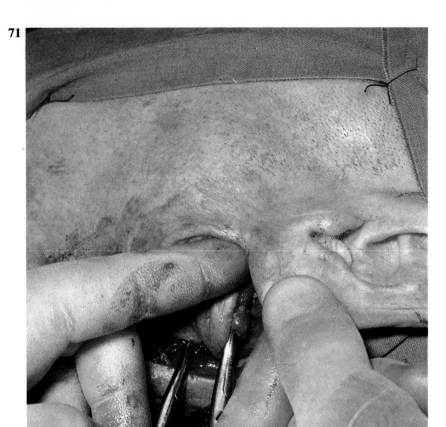

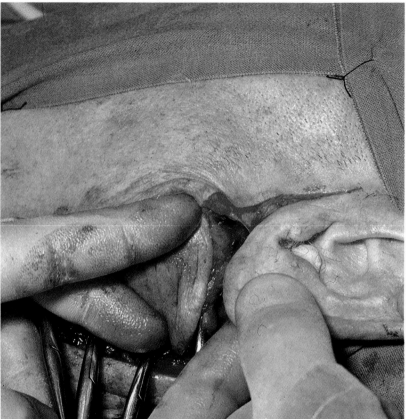

71 The surgeon now prepares to make the facial part of the cervico-mastoid-facial incision. His left index finger is pushing the lump forwards, while the pinna is being held backwards so that again the knife can make the incision in the skin crease in front of the ear without cutting into the tumour. Note the cotton-wool plug in the ear.

72 The facial part of the incision has been made right up to the zygoma, and deepened through the superficial fascia. The posterior margin of the tumour is bulging the parotid tissue backwards just behind the surgeon's left index finger, but the combination of pushing the !ump forwards and pulling the pinna backwards has permitted the incision to be made safely without cutting into the tumour.

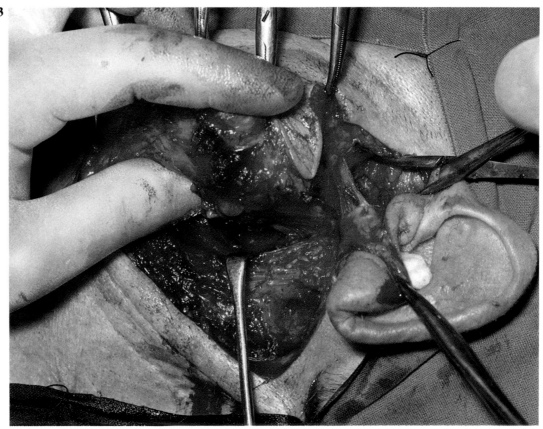

73 **The natural plane of cleavage between the parotid anteriorly and the cartilage of the external auditory meatus posteriorly has been opened up** as shown by the pair of opened artery forceps, and the space in front of the three muscles in the cervical part of the incision is demonstrated with the aid of the retractor. Between these two cavities lies the bridge of tissue which now has to be whittled away to expose the facial nerve trunk and bifurcation.

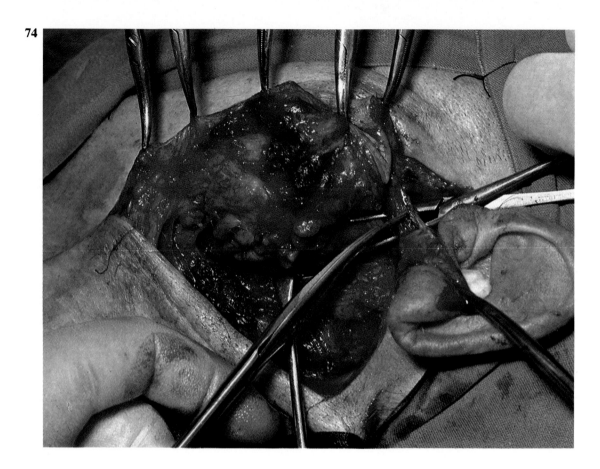

74 Process of whittling away the bridge of tissues between the two cavities. A pair of artery forceps is pushed through the bridge at the depth of 1mm or 2mm so that its points emerge at the lower border of the bridge, and this isolated piece of the bridge is divided with scissors.

75 The bridge has been completely whittled away to expose the trunk of the facial nerve and its bifurcation. The dissecting forceps touches the trunk of the nerve at its bifurcation, while the retractor holds down the anterior border of the sternomastoid muscle and the posterior belly of the digastric. The stylohyoid has not been included in the pull of the retractor.

It will be clear that the lump (the surgeon's left thumb is resting on it) is closely applied to the upper division of the nerve and it would seem that any attempt to dissect the upper division of the nerve at this stage might involve a definite chance of breaching the capsule of the tumour. Therefore, it was decided to expose the lowermost branch of the lower division and then work upwards serially along the various branches of the facial nerve from below upwards, turning the superficial parotid with its enclosed tumour upwards from below, instead of forwards from behind.

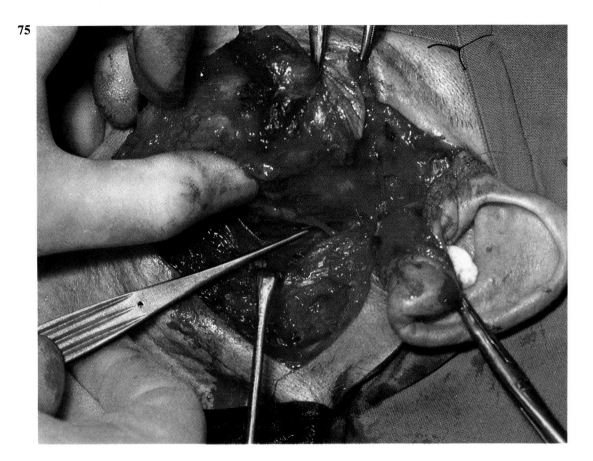
75

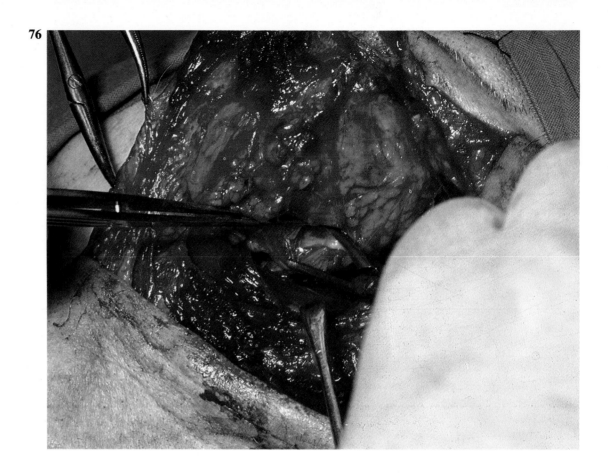

76 Lower division of the facial nerve being dissected forwards with emphasis on lowermost branch. The artery forceps have been pushed along just superficial to the nerve and the tissues between the split blades have been divided with a pair of scissors.

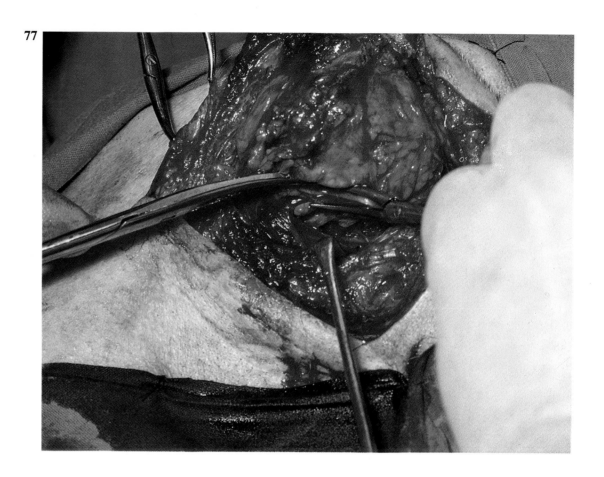

77 **Dissection of the lowermost branch of the lower division** continues
and rather more of the nerve has been exposed at this stage.

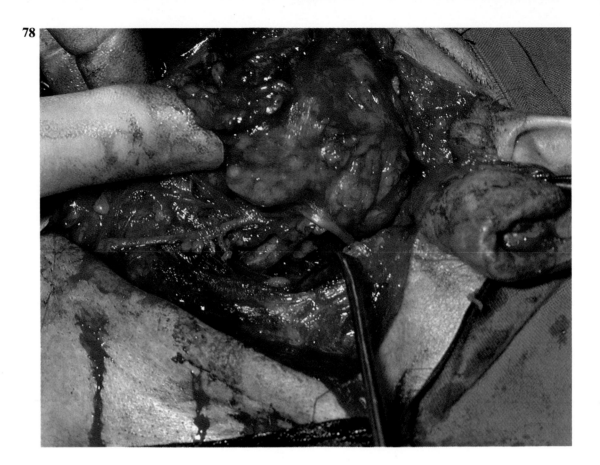

78 **The whole of the lowermost branch of the lower division, that is the platysmal branch, has been demonstrated right up to the margin of the skin incision.** The next branch, the mandibular branch, is also now visible approaching the operator's left thumb. That thumb is pushing the mass upwards and away from the facial nerve and the dissector. Note the lobulated tumour mass at the region to which the left thumb points, and also immediately above the trunk of the facial nerve. There is still a thin layer of connective tissue overlying the lobulated tumour, but it is easy to see how the mass overhangs the bifurcation of the nerve and particularly its upper division.

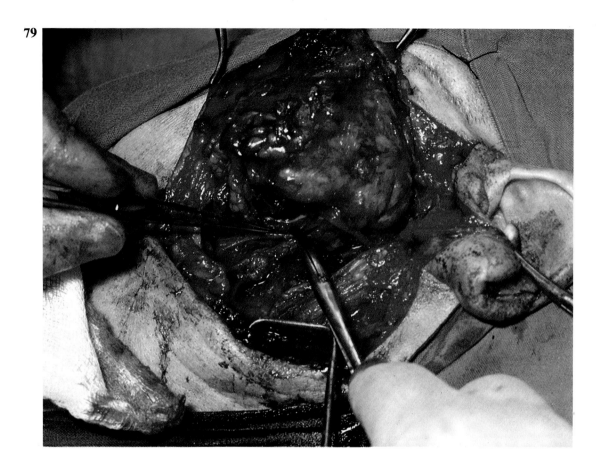

79 Lower buccal branch exposed. The dissecting forceps in the surgeon's left hand points at the mandibular branch of the facial nerve, and the lower buccal branch is now visible in front of that nerve and is to be dissected away from the superficial parotid with its contained tumour.

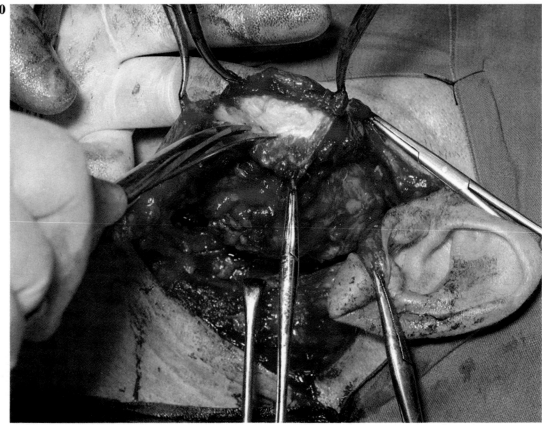

80 Raising of skin-flap. At this stage it became clear that, even with this technique, the further dissection of the branches of the upper division of the facial nerve would be hazardous, because of the way they were completely overlain by the tumour mass. Because it was quite clear that the mass was superficial to all the nerve branches, it was deemed safe at this stage to reflect the skin-flap in the hope that this would give greater mobility of the superficial parotid and make the remaining dissection technically easier. The skin-flap is being raised in the plane of yellow subcutaneous fat immediately superficial to the superficial part of the parotid salivary gland.

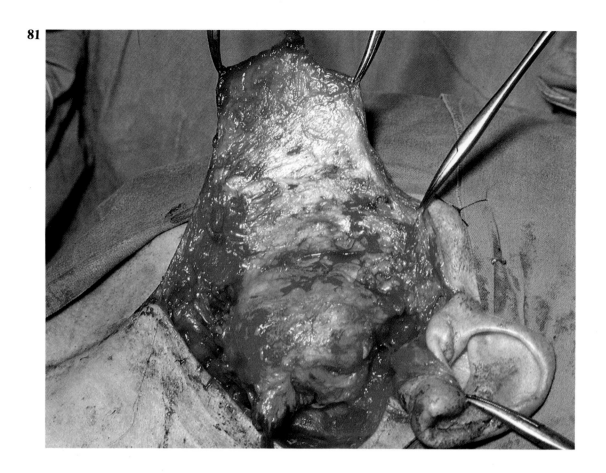

81   The raising of the skin-flap is complete and one now sees exposed the whole of the superficial parotid with its enclosed tumour, not visible from this angle except as a bulge.

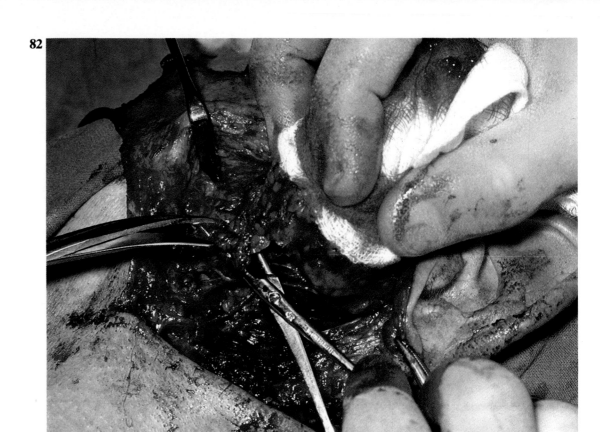

82 Dissection of lower buccal branch. With the aid of the greater mobility obtained by the reflection of the skin-flap, the lower buccal branch is now being dissected forwards towards the region of the parotid duct, i.e. the position of the right-angled retractor. The usual combination of blunt and sharp dissection is being used.

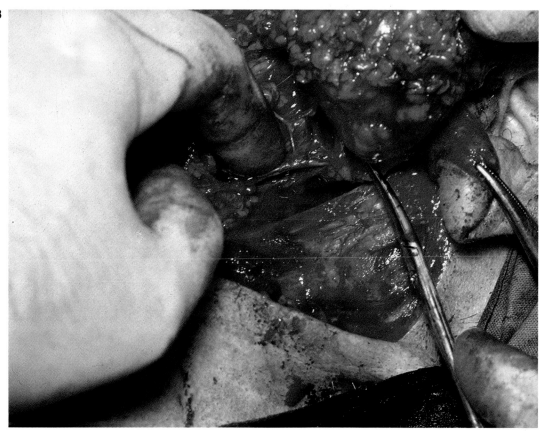

83 An upper buccal branch from the lower division of the nerve has now been demonstrated, in this view immediately to the right of the operator's left index finger. The artery forceps in the surgeon's right hand is pointing at the origin of the upper division of the nerve at the bifurcation. It is still rather overhung by the mass of tumour tissue immediately superficial to the point of the forceps, but the increased mobility of the superficial parotid has made a direct attack on the dissection of this upper division feasible.

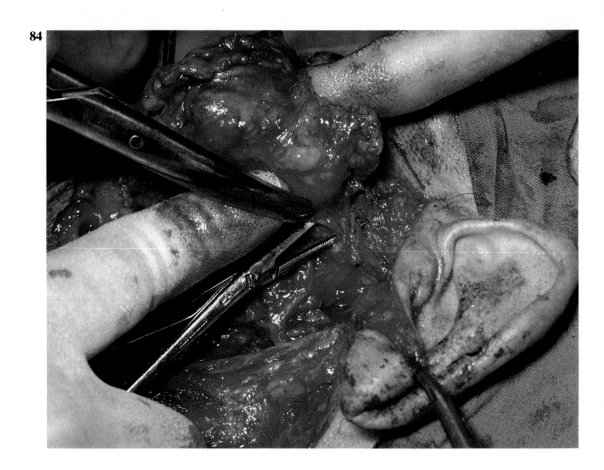

84 Dissection of the upper division of the nerve has started. Notice how the surgeon's right index finger and an assistant's index finger are gently manoeuvring the tumour and the whole superficial parotid forwards and upwards so as to permit a direct view of the dissection.

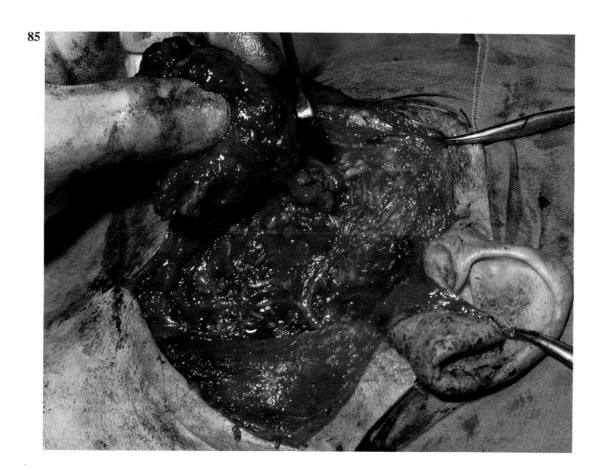

85   The uppermost branch of the upper division has been traced to the upper border of the incision as the temporal branch, and from its anterior border the zygomatic branch towards the orbit is now visible and about to be traced upwards and forwards to the anterior skin-flap, aiming at the point where the right-angled retractor rests.

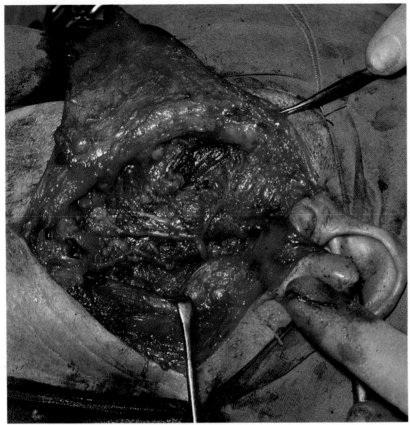

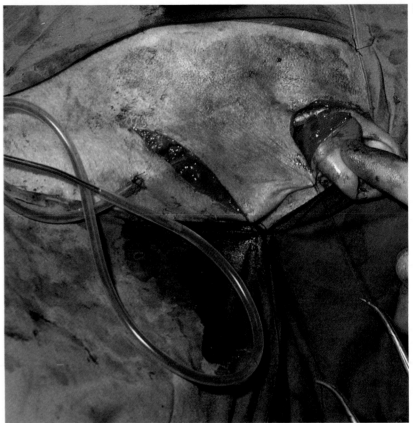

86 Removal of superficial parotid and tumour. The completion of the dissection forwards of the zygomatic branch has resulted in the complete freeing of the superficial parotid and its enclosed tumour mass. Note the masseter muscle fibres in the anterior portion of the wound where they have been exposed by the dissection of the zygomatic and upper buccal branches. In this illustration the facial nerve branches are clearly shown.

87 Stay sutures into skin-flaps. A drainage tube has been inserted from within outwards with the help of a sharp-pointed metal introducer so that the hole in the skin fits very snugly as an airtight fit around the tubing. Stay sutures have been inserted into the skin-flaps to indicate the position in which they should lie when the final suture is inserted.

88 The incision is closed with one long continuous suture using blanket stitch. This stitch gives excellent apposition at every point along the wound because of the lateral bar maintaining pressure everywhere. It is also easy to remove because, except at the ends where the stitch is knotted, the removal of the sutures is very easy after cutting the length of suture parallel to the wound. Thereby, the necessity to dig into the tender lines of the healing scar in order to divide the cross-overs is obviated.

Suction is maintained continuously by means of the Canny–Ryall syringe, a rubber bulb attached to the tubing via a plastic connector. The bulb is squeezed and connected to the tubing and then released. The suction so obtained is gentle but effective. Be careful that there is no air leak, either along the suture line (the lower border of the ear is a particularly dangerous spot) or at the hole for the drainage tube. An extra stitch or two may be required. A further aid to getting the wound airtight is to apply a liquid dressing of the type that sets to a firm skin. Whitehead's varnish is effective and has a pleasing smell! The rubber bulb must be observed closely for the first hour or so in case a leak should develop or it fills with blood. Once the bulb is full it is no longer sucking, and it must be detached from the tubing, emptied and reapplied in the collapsed position. After the first hour it is usually requested that the nursing staff empty it at hourly intervals for the first 8 hours, and then at 4 hourly intervals until a decision is made to remove the drain.

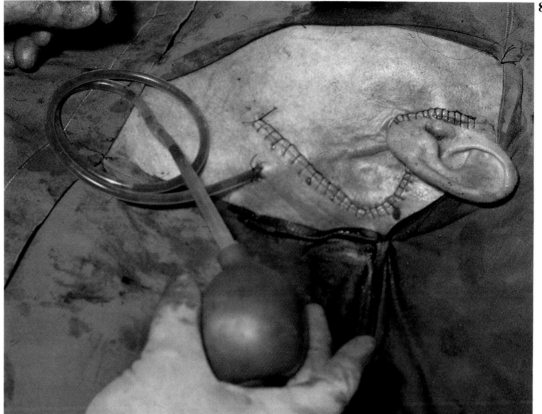

Variation if there has been a previous operation

If the surgeon is faced with a patient in whom a parotid tumour has **89** 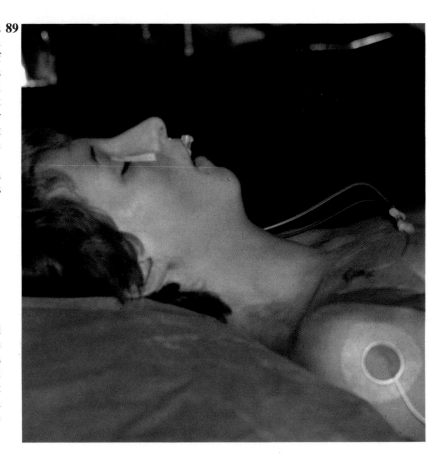 previously been excised, or in whom an attempt has been made previously to excise a parotid tumour, and the present problem is one of recurrence or residual tumour, it is important to view the previous incision as potentially containing tumour cells, even though clinical examination fails to show any such evidence. Therefore, it follows that the previous scar must be excised in continuity with the present tumour mass or masses. The necessity to do this can produce some difficult problems with regard to the modification of the incision, and even the use of local or distant skin-flaps. Each case must be considered separately. However, **89** to **98** show a few details of an operation in which a recurrence of parotid tumour was associated with the scar of a previous removal.

89 Patient anaesthetised; in this particular case an oral endotracheal tube was used. Note the protection of the eye and the presence of the electrocardiograph leads. A pillow is still present under the head: this is about to be removed and replaced with the usual head-ring. The lump and overlying scar are too inconspicuous to be easily seen in this view, but they lie immediately below the point where the lower border of the pinna meets the face. The blue mark to indicate which side of the patient is to be operated on is shown low in the neck.

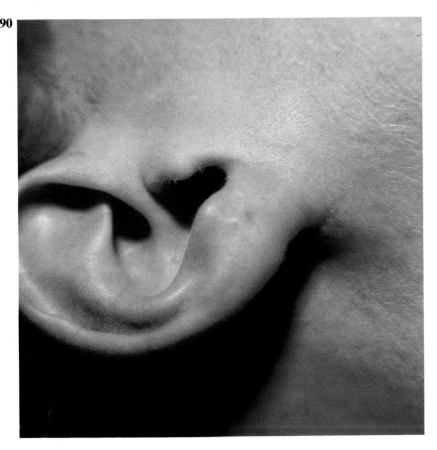

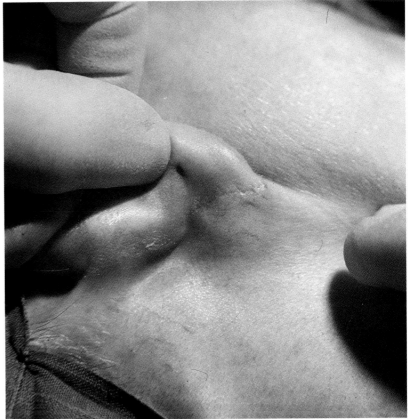

90   In close-up, the bulge of the lump below the lower border of the pinna is visible and also the scar running across it. The histology of the previous lesion in this 40-year-old woman had been a pleomorphic salivary adenoma, but the operation for its removal had been a local enucleation, a form of operation with a significant incidence of recurrence because it does not guarantee a margin of normal tissue all round the lump.

91   Lump and overlying scar. Pulling the ear lobe upwards and forwards, after cleaning the skin and towelling up, has made the lump and its overlying scar more obvious. Wounds in this region heal extremely well and sometimes it is very difficult to see the scar of a previous operation. It is also very surprising how often patients do not remember to give a history of the previous operation! Always look very closely for a scar in every patient with a parotid lump.

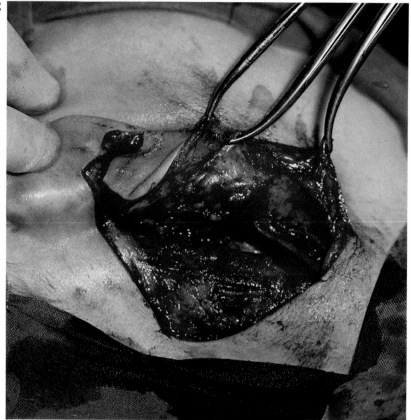

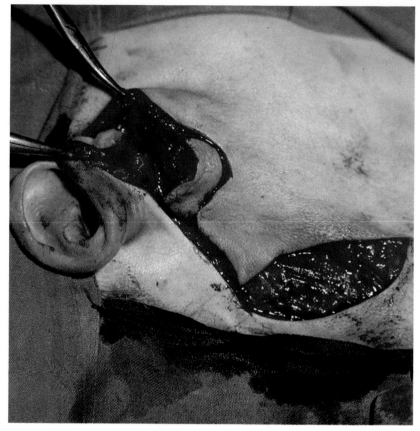

92 The whole of the cervico-mastoid-facial incision has been made, with the modification that an extra anterior loop incision has been made to circumscribe, with an oval island of skin, the scar and about 3 cm to 4 cm of tissue in all directions round it. The cervical part of the preliminary dissection has been performed, and the sternomastoid and posterior belly of the digastric muscles are clearly seen, although the overhanging parotid tissue obscures the stylohyoid muscle. Note, that in order to take the posterior part of the mastoid incision clear of the old scar, it has been necessary to site it on the posterior surface of the pinna.

93 Deepening facial wound. This view shows clearly the facial part of the preliminary dissection in which the natural plane of cleavage between the parotid salivary gland anteriorly and the cartilage of the external auditory meatus posteriorly has been deepened down to the commencement of the bony external auditory meatus. Note the island of skin around the old scar.

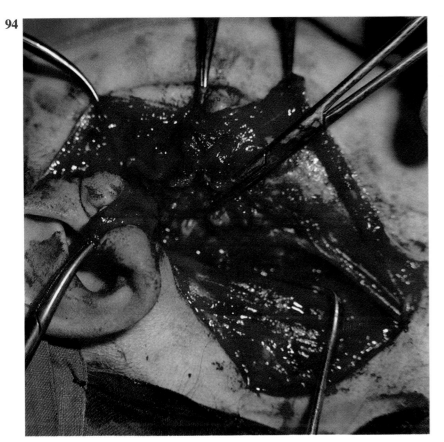

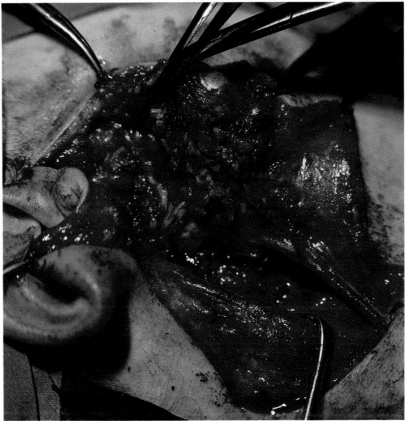

94 Exposure of trunk and bifurcation of facial nerve. The bridge of tissues between the upper and lower dissections has been divided to expose the trunk and bifurcation of the facial nerve. The artery forceps in the centre of the picture is pointing at the nerve. Notice that the direction in which the nerve is running is almost directly forwards, rather than forwards and downwards as it has appeared in previous illustrations. The reason for this was the tissue deformity produced by previous surgery.

95 The uppermost branch of the upper division of the facial nerve has been followed to the margin of the skin incision.

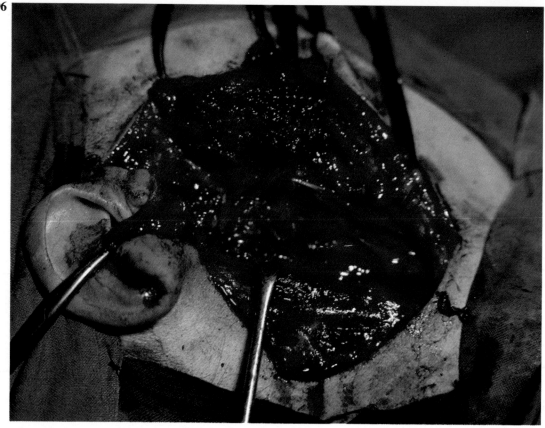

96　Lowermost branch of the lower division has been dissected forwards.
In the region where it passes the external jugular vein, the branch which
ultimately will reach the angle of the mouth, the mandibular branch, is
clearly seen. When the lowermost (platysmal) branch has been
completely followed to the margin of the skin incision, it will be time to
reflect the skin-flap.

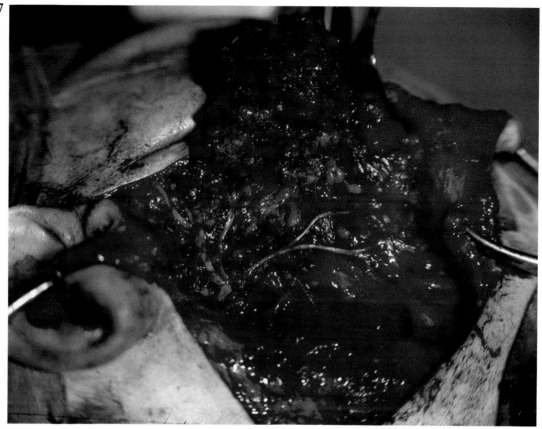

97 Reflection of the anterior skin-flap has started. The superficial part of the parotid has been dissected off the trunk and branches of the facial nerve almost to the anterior border of the salivary gland, and the recurrent mass of tumour within the parotid cannot be seen on this deep surface of the superficial part of the parotid salivary gland.

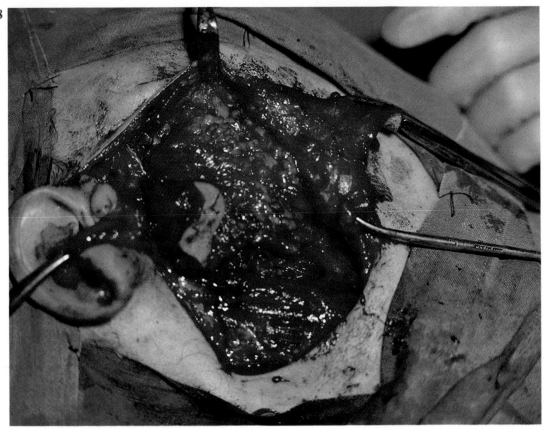

98 The same structures as in the previous illustration (97) are shown here, but with the superficial part of the parotid salivary gland allowed to fall backwards over the facial nerve and its branches, so that the island of skin, which is about to be excised in continuity with the superficial part of the gland and its contained tumour, can be seen clearly. The dissection will be completed by demonstrating the most anterior parts of the courses of the branches of the facial nerve at the anterior margin of the gland, thereby detaching the superficial parotid and completing the superficial conservative parotidectomy.

Other parotidectomy operations

No further consideration will be given to parotidectomy as part of a more major procedure, involving for example block dissection of the neck, resection of the jaw and pinna and zygoma. In such operations the parotidectomy is a minor part of the whole procedure and there is no question of any attempt at conserving the facial nerve.

With regard to semi-conservative and radical parotidectomy without any larger excision of neighbouring tissues, the key to the surgeon's decision to sacrifice the trunk or a branch of the facial nerve depends upon his judgment whether he can safely dissect the nerve off the lump without cutting into the lump. An important aid in making this decision is whether the nerve seems to be pushed aside by the presence of the lump and altered in its course by it, or whether it keeps running on straight into the lump. This sort of decision is the most difficult one that a surgeon performing a parotidectomy has to take. It is the author's advice that until he develops enough experience to be happy to make up his own mind on difficult questions like this, he errs on the side of sacrificing a branch of the facial nerve rather than getting too close to the tumour. Destruction of one branch of the facial nerve rarely leads to any permanent disability of the facial muscles. The most difficult situation is of course where the whole trunk of the nerve seems to be running into the tumour. In these circumstances it might be advisable to try to find the branches of the nerve anteriorly and trace them backwards, because the relationship of the lump to the nerve may appear quite different when the tissues have been mobilised by this manoeuvre. In the last resort, however, it is important that the surgeon should have the courage to sacrifice the whole facial nerve if necessary. It follows that every patient before parotidectomy, even for what seems a small and superficial lump, should be warned that it might be necessary to sacrifice the facial nerve. Permission to do this must always be obtained.

Complications

Reactionary haemorrhage

The incidence of bleeding into the wound during the first 24 hours after the operation is significant – in the author's experience about five per cent. To try to prevent reactionary haemorrhage, when the dissection has been completed and before sewing up commences, it is most important that the patient's position be flattened from the head-up tilt to the horizontal, and that the anaesthetist be requested to reverse any drugs that he has used to produce hypotension and to infuse liquid to expand the circulating volume. Only when the systolic blood pressure has been stable for five minutes at least at 110 mmHg, or at least at 20 mm below the patient's normal blood pressure, whichever figure is the greater, should closure begin. The suction drainage must help to prevent blocking of the drain, but despite all these precautions the formation of a large haematoma in the wound cannot always be prevented.

Treatment
Take the patient back to the operating theatre, re-anaesthetise, re-open the wound and evacuate the blood clot. Sometimes one or more bleeding points are found and must be controlled by ligature or diathermy, with due caution to avoid damage to the facial nerve. All precautions to ensure that there will be no recurrence of reactionary haemorrhage are then taken again before closure.

Facial nerve paresis

Even after all branches of the facial nerve have been seen and carefully preserved, nearly all patients have detectable weakness of the facial nerve muscles on the day after the operation, at least in one territory of the face (forehead, eyes or mouth). In many this effect is transient but a very few patients have detectable weakness for up to two years. The median time of detectable weakness is about nine months. Recovery, in the author's experience, is always complete if all named branches of the nerve have been preserved. The management of the temporary paresis is mainly reassurance about prognosis, although eye drops, and even occasionally a lateral tarsorrhaphy, are appropriate to reduce conjunctival irritation.

After semi-conservative parotidectomy, it is surprising how many patients achieve a complete recovery of function of the facial muscles provided only one or two named branches have been cut.

The long-term management of complete and permanent facial nerve palsy after radical parotidectomy is outside the scope of this book.

Fistula formation

If the author's recommendations that as much as possible of the superficial parotid is excised in a superficial parotidectomy, that deep parotidectomy is always accompanied by superficial parotidectomy, and that a good length of main duct be excised with the superficial parotid, are all adopted, then the incidence of fistula should be well under one per cent. This is just as well because treatment of a fistula is very difficult: further parotidectomy puts the facial nerve at great risk, while even large doses of radiotherapy do not always result in permanent destruction of the secreting elements of the gland.

Sloughing of skin-flap

Because of the excellent blood supply of the skin of the face and neck, this complication is rare. The most likely site is the summit of the curve of the mastoid part of the incision. Treatment is along the normal lines of debridement, excision of slough and skin-grafting if necessary.

Infection

This, in the absence of sloughing of the skin-flap, is a rare complication.

Keloid

The mastoid part of the scar is often heaped up and broadened, but fortunately lies inconspicuous within the hairline.

Index

All numbers indicate page numbers.

External auditory meatus, see Meatus, external auditory
Eyes, protection of with tape   12, 64

F

Facial nerve, see Nerve, facial
Fistula, parotid   7, 44
Fossa, tonsillar   9

H

Halothane   11
Head-ring   84
Hypotension, induced   62

I

Incision for parotidectomy   15, 86
– cervical part of   15, 64, 66
– facial part of   21, 22, 23, 68
– mastoid part of 18, 66, 67
Intubation, endotracheal   11, 12, 84

J

Janes, R.M.   6

K

Keloid   14

L

Ligament, stylomandibular   50, 59

M

Mandible   14, 15, 57
– angle of   50, 64
– ramus of   54, 56
– resection of   91
Masseter muscle, see Muscle, masseter
Mastoid process, see Process, mastoid
Meatus, external auditory   13
– bone of   27, 28
– cartilage of   23, 25, 27, 28, 31, 69, 86
Monomorphic salivary adenoma   8
Muscle, buccinator   7
Muscle, digastric, posterior belly of   17, 20, 21, 28, 48, 61, 66, 67, 71, 86
Muscle, masseter   12, 38, 82
Muscle, pterygoid   58
Muscle, sternomastoid   17, 19, 20, 21, 28, 48, 56, 61, 64, 66, 67, 71, 86
Muscle, stylohyoid   17, 20, 21, 28, 48, 66, 67, 71

N

Nerve, facial   7
– bifurcation of   30, 31, 45, 71, 74, 87
– branches of: 45, 61
– – lower buccal   7, 35, 75, 78
– – mandibular   7, 41, 42, 74, 75, 88
– – platysmal   7, 35, 74, 75, 88